Firm Up All Over

Other titles in this series:

The SunSlimmer: Fight Fat, Fight Fatigue: Energy Makeover
The SunSlimmer: Fight Fat, Fight Fatigue: Diet and Cookbook

THE *SūnSlimmer*

Fight Fat, Fight Fatigue: Firm Up All Over

Nicki Waterman

Thorsons

Thorsons
An Imprint of HarperCollins*Publishers*
77–85 Fulham Palace Road
Hammersmith, London W6 8JB

The Thorsons website address is: www.thorsons.com

and *Thorsons*
are trademarks of
HarperCollins*Publishers* Limited

Published by Thorsons 2002

10 9 8 7 6 5 4 3 2 1

Sun © News Group Newspapers Ltd.

© Nicki Waterman 2002

Nicki Waterman asserts the moral right to be
identified as the author of this work

A catalogue record for this book
is available from the British Library

ISBN 0 00 711868 6

Photography by Robin Matthews

Printed and bound in Great Britain by
Martins the Printers Ltd, Berwick upon Tweed

CONTENTS

INTRODUCTION

I know what you're thinking: 'What does somebody like Nicki Waterman know about being overweight and unfit? Besides, didn't I read somewhere that all those personal trainers work out 19 hours a day and live on rice cakes? How can I possibly look like that and have a life?'

OK, let me set the record straight. *I used to be fat and lazy!*

If I could change my ways, so can you. It might seem impossible if you are overweight, totally out of shape and always breathless and tired to change, and to change quite fast – but truly, it's not. It does take some work, yes; it does take a certain amount of sticking to a routine, but it is possible to change the way you look completely; to change fat and flabby – *to fit and fantastic!*

If someone tried to tell me when I was 11½ stone (73 kg) that fitness and staying in shape would be this much fun today, I probably would have laughed. If you want the truth, I never thought I had the willpower to succeed. Sixteen years later I'm writing this book to tell you it's true and to show you how easy it is to get in shape, regardless of the body you have now.

All you have to do is make up your mind and start! You can make a start now, by reading this book. When you've done that, come back to the beginning, take a red pen and mark the things that strike a chord, the things you want to achieve and *the exercises you want to do in the first week*. It's your book – make notes anywhere you want, underline whatever you want.

After even just one week you will have more energy, working out will seem easier and you will look forward to it – it won't seem a chore. Combined with a sensible diet (for help with this you could look at another book in this series: *Fight Fat, Fight Fatigue: Energy Makeover*), not only will the weight fall off, and stay off, but you will look wonderful. If you can do it for a week, you can do it for another week.

- You'll feel (and look) firmer in as little as a week, results guaranteed.
- It is possible to completely change your body without cutting back on calories.
- Whatever your weight when you start this programme, if you have never trained before, in three months you will be firmer than you've ever been, trimmer than you've ever been and, more importantly, fitter than you've ever been.

This is no quick-fix gimmick, but you will see a noticeable difference. If you follow the directions in this book it is a recipe to a new you. I can even help you achieve this with little or no equipment. So you don't have the excuse that you can't afford expensive treadmills or stacks of weights or a personal trainer. You do have a personal trainer – me!

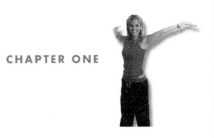

CHAPTER ONE

A BODY TO LIVE FOR –
not to die for

Take a good look at yourself in the mirror. Remember, you cannot change your bone struc-ture. Your body shape is what you have to accept as your basic frame. Then there's your natural fat and muscle ratio, the one your genes have given you. Beyond that, it's up to you.

OK – I won't deny that with dieting alone you can lose every scrap of that fat (but also muscle) if you quite literally starve yourself into a skeleton. You'll also lose your heart muscle, starve your body of essential nutrients and might even end up dead. So let's be sensible. I want you to live and I want you to live healthily. I want you to be in control of your body, not have your body in control of you.

Fat is fat and flab is flab. With the right exercise programme you can get rid of the one and tone up the other. That is what I am aiming to help you with. If you're a large woman with a big frame, you're never going to look fragile; if you're a very petite woman, you're probably never going to look like an Olympic swimmer – but what you can look is terrific!

IF I CAN DO IT, SO CAN YOU…

Before I discovered the secret of good health and fitness, I was 11½ stone (73 kg) and really out of shape for a small-framed 5'3" woman. Understandably I was daunted by the task that lay ahead of me! It was a vicious circle, and I didn't know where to start. I'd tried all sorts of silly diets because I wanted fast results – but I always ended up the same or even heavier. Now, of course, I know that the whole way I went about it was wrong, but back then I just wasn't aware.

This yo-yo effect of weight on, weight off is very like the so-called 'streaky bacon syndrome'. You're fat, lean, fat, lean – and besides being a very unflattering comparison, this approach to dieting will see you drained of energy and vitality in the long term.

This diet-binge-diet pattern can also kick-start the body into another syndrome – the camel syndrome. This is where the body (especially a woman's body) learns to store fat if it's constantly starved. It's genetic, triggered by nature to ensure against times of famine. No wonder people say that each time they go on a 'starvation' diet they end up fatter. They do! It's nature's way of looking after us.

These days, life has certainly changed for me. Becoming educated in health and fitness has helped me maintain my figure at 7½ stone (48 kg) for the past 12 years. When I reflect, I can see all too clearly why I used to struggle with my weight.

I was overweight as a teenager and enjoyed massive meals with my family, unfortunately at the expense of my waistline. When I left school I went into dentistry. The job was so sedentary I just continued to put on weight. However, it was really my actions when I was pregnant which caused my figure to expand: I ate for two when I was expecting my daughter, Alex, who is now 17. I really thought that my excess pounds would drop off after I'd given birth, but I was mistaken. It was the same for my son, Harry. Six months after he was born I was still wearing maternity clothes and people were coming up asking when my baby was due!

My Turning Point

The turning point came for me when I took time off work to look after the babies. I realized how much my confidence was affected by my weight and decided to take steps to change things, this time for good.

I teamed up with a friend who also wanted to shape up and we booked a personal trainer. Once I took that first step there was no looking back. My friend and I hit it off with our trainer, Brian, who made both the cardiovascular and weight-training sessions fun and interesting, so much so that I even did the odd one or two extra sessions on my own.

It was fun. It was working. I started to get my figure and my confidence back, I felt energized and alive, and that became my motivation.

It's a common misconception that resistance training bulks you out and prevents you from losing weight. In fact, you need to build muscle to increase your metabolism – the rate at which your body burns calories.

The more lean body tissue you have, the more calories you'll use. It's the key to success.

In addition to my exercise programme, I got to grips with two of my passions: alcohol and chocolate. I don't mean I was a heavy drinker, I just enjoyed going out socially or eating a meal with the family, and that always involved a drink – usually half a bottle of wine in the evenings and a full bottle on the weekend. I've never been much of a beer drinker, but I did enjoy the odd Scotch. These days, I will occasionally sip a white wine spritzer. That, or a diet Coke, will give me just as much of a buzz as half a bottle of wine ever did.

Due to my background in dentistry, I was already fairly well versed in nutrition, but still found some bad habits to stamp on, such as skipping breakfast. By the time you wake up in the morning your body probably has been fasting for some eight to ten hours. Your sugar levels will be low and if you don't eat a sensible breakfast, as I never did, you'll crave quick-fix snacks. I now tuck into a bowl of cereal or porridge every morning, which gives me a vital energy boost and prevents me needing high-fat snacks during the day.

Really, my eating plan hits the middle ground. I don't believe in extremes. It's important that any diet is healthy and easily maintained, especially if you have a busy job and a family. I still eat chocolate, but certainly not every day. I make sure I eat regular meals and, yes, I eat snacks throughout the day too. They're simple, high-carbohydrate, high-vitamin things like cereal and fruit, which contain carbs to help fuel my muscles for exercise.

The very best kind of diet for health and to help achieve your ideal weight is the one in the companion book to this one, *Fight Fat, Fight Fatigue: Energy Makeover*. It reveals all the nutrients you need for good health and is packed with delicious recipes too.

But it's no good following a healthier diet if the most exercise you get during the week is walking to your car, driving to work and sitting at a desk all day, then flopping on that couch in the evening to watch TV. If you want to be slim and healthy you must burn up those calories and the only way to do that is to get moving. It doesn't matter if the way you do that is to run up and down the stairs for half an hour, go for a power walk, swim 20 lengths or weight-train. Whatever suits your lifestyle and whatever you will do regularly is what works for you.

How I Started

When I started training, like everyone else once they bite the bullet and make that effort, I was eager to be slim, fit and lithe inside 24 hours, but I had to be realistic. I was 60 per cent above my ideal body weight, so I knew it would take time to achieve really noticeable results safely. Losing too much weight too fast is dangerous, so although some of the body changes brought about by exercise showed quickly, the total change I sought was by no means rapid.

I got a lot of enjoyment out of the sessions and accepted that I would have to be patient to achieve my perfect figure. However, even a few pounds off shows on the face, the ankles and the hands, while toning does make a difference all over. I soon discovered that exercise does make a difference to your shape. Think of your lungs like the carburettor of a car – the extra oxygen you take in while exercising does make you more vital and alert, which helps you want to keep going and burns off those calories.

It was great when people came up to me and commented on how good I looked. In two years, not only had I dropped all my excess flab to get down to a healthy weight, but I had also completely changed my shape and my energy levels were amazingly high. I never stopped!

I had thought, too, that once I got to my desired weight it would sort of plateau out, but I have noticed that after several years my body shape is still getting better; if anything, I feel as if it is constantly rejuvenating itself, almost as if I am pushing back the clock.

In fact, I did so well, Brian, our personal trainer, encouraged me to do all the necessary courses to qualify as a personal trainer myself.

Still, the years of unsuccessful dieting are all too fresh in my mind and my empathy for those who are struggling with their weight prompts hundreds of letters a week from men and women who are unhappy with their size. Because I know what people are going through when they're slimming, I've made sure that my approach to weight loss – sensible healthy eating and exercise – is straightforward and attainable for everyone.

PATIENCE MAKES PERFECT

First things first. Here is some scientific information to absorb to help you understand what goes on when you get locked into a diet-binge cycle without a proper exercise programme.

If you have battled with a weight problem your entire life, don't expect things to change overnight. Studies show that continual dieting which results in weight-loss which is then regained may make your ultimate, successful weight-loss more difficult to achieve. Continually dieting to lose weight, without exercising, affects muscle mass. With each successive diet the body loses more muscle mass. Even if you gain and lose the same 2 stone, the ratio of fat to muscle in your body changes. The amount of fat you're carrying increases. As time goes on, this higher percentage of body fat causes your body to slow down and use fewer calories for energy. Thus, even though you are eating the same amount of food, more of it is now turning to fat. The result is you continue to gain back more 'fat' weight with each successive diet.

The good news is that an exercise programme can stop this rebound effect. By building back the lean muscle tissue, the body's metabolism will change, although it may take your body some months to begin to use calories efficiently again.

Patience is something I have learned through my years of training, especially when it comes to improving the shape of my butt! I can spend hours squatting and lunging, because I know that each individual squat or lunge brings me one step closer to the 'perfect' rear. It's the sum of each repetition that eventually creates the ultimate result. The same principle applies to your body and physical fitness. If you expect overnight results, you're setting yourself up for disappointment. When I started training, there were times when I would get frustrated because I was working so hard and, although there were definite improvements, I still hadn't achieved the shape I was ultimately aiming for.

Then, one day, everything seemed to fall into place. But it wasn't just a few lucky workouts that got me there. It was the sum of all my workouts put together – over nearly a year – that had gradually made the difference.

Whenever I get impatient and want to see results faster, I think of how much I achieved when I first started. Each workout is loads of reps and sets bringing me one step closer to my desired results. It will be the same for you. Work hard and be consistent and you can expect change in direct proportion to your time and effort. The extra specially brilliant news is that people who haven't exercised properly before get brilliant results quickly.

HOW TO GET AND STAY ON A ROLL

Have you ever tried to start riding a bike uphill? It's pretty hard to get going from a stationary position, isn't it? It's the same with an exercise programme. Once you get a bit of momentum going, you'll find what seemed like an uphill struggle becomes an achievable goal.

The more you exercise, the more energy you will have, the more results you'll see and the more motivated you'll be to keep going.

Once you start exercising and eating right, you've smashed the sluggishness and are on a roll ... hopefully a permanent one – like for the rest of your life!

Remember, it's that sluggishness, that lack of inactivity, that has helped pile on the flab in the first place.

7

So, don't delay, don't resist and don't be afraid of the perceived costs of success or you'll remain stuck and stationary. Just jump in. Get on a roll. Any way you do it, once you gain momentum, you're halfway there.

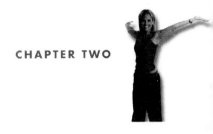

CHAPTER TWO

GAINING THE UPPER HAND

Much of how we control our attitudes, moods and feelings comes from how we feel about ourselves. Life can be a roller-coaster if you let it. One moment you're up, the next down. Up, down, up, down – it's pretty scary and unpredictable.

Positive people who feel good about themselves can often turn a negative situation into a positive one, or at least survive the experience without being devastated.

The key is to gain control from the inside out.

What does that really mean? Accepting yourself for starters – and getting in shape is the first step. Whatever they say, no one really wants to be fat and flabby and tired all the time. Not only is the lack of 'get up and go' demoralizing, but, quite literally, it's unhealthy, leading to many illnesses and medical problems. Self-image and self-respect are zero. Depression can set in.

Those who dwell on negatives or failure are often fearful and lacking in confidence. A negative attitude not only erodes your sense of control and purpose, but also chisels away at your sense of inner worth, resulting in low self-esteem which can stop you from realizing your potential. So be positive, realistic and go for it.

Tell yourself you're worth the effort. You deserve fitness and energy. Don't retreat into your inner secret self, treating it as separate from your outer self, thinking the outer part counts for nothing. Both parts are you – and all of you counts. So grab yourself back, take control. Get in shape. It will change the way you feel about yourself as well as your mental outlook – not just about yourself, but about everything around you.

Suddenly, you're glowing. It's like a contagious energy, something you wish you could bottle and share with others. You're positive, things look good – inside and out, you're happy! Isn't that worth working for?

LET GO OF GUILT

Nobody's perfect, not even those fashion models on magazine covers. (Ever heard of air brushing? It not only removes wrinkles, but sometimes lots of pounds too!)

If you've ever pigged-out, missed a workout or caught yourself acting like a couch potato, you know how powerful the guilt can be. You didn't live up to your expectations and you feel you've let yourself down.

Guilt can take over, inhibiting your actions and destroying your self-confidence and self-respect. Ultimately, guilt can be just as destructive as a physical illness. Like a downhill snowball that picks up more and more snow, guilt gets bigger and bigger until it flattens you. There you are, right at the bottom of the slope with this giant mountain of guilt sitting on top of you, powerless and unable to pick yourself up. You feel negative not only about the 'bad' thing you did, but about yourself in general. Talk about making a mountain out of a molehill!

People have different ways of dealing with guilt where their exercise programme is concerned. Some get stuck and can't move, others go into a blind frenzy and exercise until they're ready to drop, but inwardly, they feel angry the entire time. Both extremes are unhealthy. Before succumbing to guilt, ask yourself where it's getting you. Is there anything redeeming about the guilt or is it just a colossal waste of your time and energy?

Remember: you are human and there is always room for error.

Missing a workout is not the end of the world. Learn to laugh at your defeats and use them as learning experiences. Reframe the negative into a positive. Meanwhile, console yourself with these three workout facts:

1   Accomplishing 15 per cent of a workout is better than doing nothing at all. Can't bear the thought of power walking for half an hour? Do 10 minutes (and I bet you get so energized you do the whole thing anyway!)
2   Don't wait for things to be perfect to start. You may wait for the rest of your life. For instance, 'Oh, I'll start this workout after I answer all my telephone calls, or after I've washed the dishes.' There are always things we need to do. Make working out a priority, not an afterthought. Do it first – then do your chores. You'll even find your chores are easier.
3   Set realistic goals. Don't expect perfection – just the best you can realistically be. Make that your goal, not conforming to the ideal set out by some model on a magazine cover. If your goal is set too high, you'll end up using it as an excuse not to start in the first place.

HOW TO SET GOALS

Your fitness goals must be established after a sensible assessment of what you can realistically accomplish for yourself. It is helpful to look through magazines and other media for pictures of people with similar body types to yours (see pages 137–51). Examine what they have accomplished. If you are short and naturally curvaceous like me, look at the changes Janet Jackson, Jennifer Lopez and Madonna have made to their bodies. There's no point in wanting to be like Kate Moss or Denise Lewis if they are not your body type. When you've found the image you want, use it as your guide – but be certain the person is similar to you in height, build, bone structure, age and fat-accumulation areas. Madonna is only four years older than me and looks amazing. While I was losing weight I had a picture of her on my fridge door to act as a constant reminder of what I could achieve. Why don't you cut out a photo of a possible role model and use it for motivation?

You also have to create a clear mental picture of what you want to achieve. This will help you reach your fitness goals. Close your eyes for a second and visualize yourself in peak shape, then envision doing physical activities you really love. Finally, what have you always dreamed of doing that getting in great shape would finally let you do?

Here are seven rules that can help you turn goals into reality:

Seven Rules for Turning your Goals into Reality

1 **Set Goals with a Reason in Mind**

Your ultimate goal must surely be happiness. Let's say you want to lose 10 lb. Ask yourself why. Because your clothes will fit better? Because you'll feel better about yourself? Because you'll be healthier and live longer? Maybe your reasons are one or all of the above. If you know what they are before you get started, your motivation will automatically build. Would you start a long drive without knowing your destination? Of course not. Set goals that are backed by your own strong desire.

2 **Do It for Yourself**

Not for your boyfriend, husband, mother-in-law, distant cousin … *for yourself*. While advice from family and friends is fine, if you don't really want it their advice will sound like nagging and we all know what we do when someone nags us: nothing!

3 **Accept Responsibility for Achieving your Goal**

Go ahead, own it. It's yours, so set up a game plan and get moving. Take that first step and you'll put yourself in the right frame of mind to achieve your goal. Remember – think positive. You're a winner. Go for your goal 100 per cent. It's all about trying, so don't give up!

4 **Give Yourself a Concrete but Realistic Deadline**

Let's face it. If we had forever to get in shape, it would probably take that long. But we don't have forever; we only have now. Setting a deadline will work like a kick in the backside to jump-start you into action. By creating a sense of urgency, due dates can help prevent you from coming up with endless excuses. And if you're anything like me, you probably have a million of them already lined up. If your ultimate goal is to lose 4 stone, break it into mini-goals with mini-deadlines. For instance, plan to lose 2 lb the first week and 8 lb by the end of the first month. This is a safe and realistic goal, which sounds a lot easier than losing all 4 stone and shape up at once. Also, not only is it easier to foresee losing half a stone at a time, rather than 4 in one fell swoop, but you can reward yourself along the way and use the thrill of those step-by-step victories to keep losing more until you achieve your final goal. Achieving many small goals will fortify you for the long haul. It's like giving yourself a pat on the back to keep motivated.

5 **Develop a Plan of Attack**

How do you plan to reach those goals and what steps will get you there? Also, what are you willing to put up with or do without to get there? If you want to lose half a stone, you must step up your activity and eat less, or maybe change your eating patterns. If you're currently a couch potato, that means exercising three or four times a week for at least 20 minutes at a stretch. Work out where you can take that time for those sessions from your week and fit them in. When I have an all-day photo shoot or I'm filming for a TV show, my time for training is really crunched, so I simply get up half an hour earlier and work out then. Does it work? I can guarantee it does. Twenty minutes is really very little. Look at your phone bill to calculate how long you spend chatting to friends on the phone, or perhaps how long you spend reading magazines. You'll be surprised at how time mounts up. Use some of that time for exercising instead. We all have 'lost' minutes we can spare – so be honest! You know where your lost minutes are. Decide what

13

steps are necessary to reach your goals. Then work out how you're going to follow through.

6 Get It Down on Paper

It's essential to write your goals down. That way, they're permanent and there's no chance of changing them. The list can also be a great visual tool! Try writing your goals in two-foot-high letters and hang them somewhere where you'll see them every day. Or stick reminders on your bathroom mirror or on the fridge. If you really want your goals to be embedded in your memory for life, mimic those old school teachers and force yourself to write them down over and over and over, until you could write them in your sleep.

7 Leave Room for Obstacles and Opportunities

Life usually doesn't flow in a straight line, so don't set yourself up for a foolproof journey from fat to fit. Anticipate detours, obstacles – even total mess-ups and pig-outs, but don't let them burn you out or derail you. Just pick yourself up, dust yourself off and press on!

For example, I suffered a knee injury while training for the 1995 London Marathon. I could have given up and not entered that year, but I had been working toward that goal for months and hated to throw in the towel. So rather than changing my goal, I changed the direction of my workout programme to focus on different body parts, until I could use my legs again. Guess what happened? That year, I finished in 3 hours 36 minutes, and came in the top 400 women out of 35,000!

The pessimist sees the half-glass of water as half empty; the optimist as half full. It's still the same old half-glass of water. The only difference is how you perceive it. So embrace those detours, because who knows? Sometimes detours lead you to less obvious solutions than you ever would have discovered had you stuck to the main route.

SUMMING UP

OK, guys and girls, start your engines. Put aside your fear, because fear leads to failure – and besides, once you get started you'll be too busy and happy to feel fear, and too motivated to stop.

Don't waste your energy dreaming up excuses. Instead, dream up goals, visualize what you really want to look like, write or draw your goals in two-foot-high letters. Most of all – keep the faith.

Think winner, not loser. Happiness, not sadness. Fit, not fat.

Make your fitness programme a game that's fun, exciting and challenging. Think of yourself as becoming fit and healthy and, before you know it, you will be! Don't look back, complain or feel sorry for yourself. Be thankful for what you have and never take that for granted.

Even if you're technically overweight or obese, dwelling on how 'bad' your current position is just counterproductive and likely to lead only to doomed attempts at quick-fix dieting. And, as I've explained earlier, the only thing crash diets do is make you fatter. You'll succeed with patience and by keeping your eye on your long-term goals.

I'll repeat – you don't have to cut calories to lose weight.

But you do have to burn those excess calories up and firm up the flab, and the only way you're going to do that is by working out. Even if you've never exercised before, don't despair. In this book I'm going to teach you everything you need to know to uncover, once and for all, the beautiful body and energized person that's been hiding away.

We're in this together, so just stick with me and we'll succeed. I promise ... but give it a wholehearted chance!

15

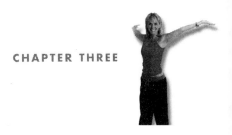

CHAPTER THREE

FIRST STEPS TO A NEW YOU

You can work on different areas of your body individually after warming up, but if you intend to do a complete workout it is recommended that you do this in the safest way. Here's a list of the different muscle groups:

17

Upper Body
Chest
Back
Shoulders
Biceps
Triceps

Lower Body
Quads
Hamstrings
Buttocks
Inner thigh
Outer thigh
Calf muscles

Core
Abs

FIRST STEPS

Your first steps are the most important; this section gives you all the information you'll need to ensure you exercise safely and get the best results from your workouts right from the start. This 'First Steps Workout' is straightforward, and will only take 10 minutes. There are four stages all in all, including the Workout, which we'll describe in detail below. Go for it!

1   The Warm-up
2   How to Breathe
3   Aerobic Exercise and Target Heart Rate
4   Your First Steps 10-minute Workout

Note: Never work the same muscle groups two days in a row, as this can cause excessive strain and possible damage.

1. THE WARM-UP

Always warm up first before training or stretching or doing aerobic exercise.

This is Rule Number 1. A gradual warm-up protects your muscles from sudden damage. Try 5 or 10 minutes of low-intensity aerobic activity, such as light running on the spot to get your heart rate up. Anything light will do, such as easy skipping, moderately fast walking, stepping or running up and down the stairs. Whatever is convenient. Don't overdo it – remember, you're only warming up, not going for the burn!

If life suddenly becomes even more hectic than usual, you can always find time to fit in your regular warm-up period. It's better than nothing at all, will stop you feeling guilty and will help you to maintain the exercise habit.

Remember: *The warm-up comes first.*

Fight Fat, Fight Fatigue

2. HOW TO BREATHE

We all breathe automatically without thought; but you would be surprised at how many people don't do it right. They take little breaths, the bare minimum, their lungs are never filled so they never get enough oxygen. It's like a car running with a blocked carburettor or fuel line. Exercise needs oxygen – and getting fit goes hand in hand with breathing well and making the best use of your lungs.

- Expand your lungs – get that oxygen in!
- Learn how to 'Open the breath'.
- Proper breathing helps you to fight stress and fatigue, boosts memory, improves endurance, relieves depression, aids digestion, lowers blood pressure, increases circulation, conquers insomnia, boosts sexual drive and speeds up metabolism – which helps burn off fat.

When they first start training with me, many of my clients are unable to take a deep, satisfying breath. I notice this when I ask them to do some power-walking, skipping, cycling and so on, so I teach them all how to 'open the breath' – taking deep, long inhalations and even longer exhalations. Their shortness of breath soon disappears. Not only does this simple technique improve endurance to help you train better, but has all the wonderful side-effects listed above. Not bad for something we have to do every day, but often don't get right.

Three Steps to Better Breathing

Practise any one of the following exercises every day and you will soon notice a positive difference.

19

EXERCISE BREATHING

When lifting weights or doing resistance work, exhale when your muscles contract and inhale on the recovery to help your body restore itself. Slow down your workout until this rhythm becomes automatic. If you're running or doing intense aerobic activity, try counting (actually mouthing numbers) when you exhale, which can train the rib cage to stay expanded for longer.

THE RELAXING BREATH

When you're feeling stressed, sit or lie down with your back straight and place the tip of your tongue on the roof of your mouth behind your teeth. Exhale completely through your mouth, then inhale through your nose for 4 seconds. Hold the breath for 7 seconds, then exhale audibly through the mouth for 8 seconds. Repeat 4 times.

THE STIMULATING BREATH

For a quick pick-me-up that you can do absolutely anywhere to boost your energy, sit with your back straight and the tip of your tongue on the roof of your mouth. Breathe in and out rapidly through your nose (3 cycles per second) with your mouth slightly closed. Do this for 15 seconds at first, working up to a minute. This is the perfect exercise if you've been at your desk for a while working or studying and feel like nodding off. You can even do it on a long drive – but remember to pull off the road first!

The Ideal Breath

The ideal breath should feel something like this: Place one hand on your stomach between your rib cage and navel, then sniff. (That thing moving is your diaphragm.) Place your other hand on your chest and concentrate on using your diaphragm to make the hand on your stomach rise higher than the hand on your chest. Extend your out-breath to twice the length of your in-breath.

3. AEROBIC EXERCISE AND TARGET HEART RATE

Aerobics – raising your oxygen levels.

Some people call it aerobics, some call it cardiovascular activity. It means getting oxygen pumping fast to where it's needed. Whatever you call it, this activity tones the heart and the vascular system (veins and arteries) and pumps oxygen around the body to raise the metabolism. A higher metabolism burns more calories and you've already read about the energizing benefits of extra oxygen.

There are two kinds of aerobics – *light* and *intense.*

Light aerobics will form part of your warm-up routine to get your heart rate up and your blood circulating around your muscles prior to training. **Intense aerobics** is a training routine in itself, which you must work up to.

THR – Target Heart Rate

Your heart beats faster when you're working harder. This means you can use a measure of your heart rate as an easy indicator of how hard or gently your body is working during exercise. When you exercise, you can use your heart rate as a guide to ensure you're working at the right pace and that you're exercising within a safe level. Working to heart rate is the ideal safe way to build aerobic capacity and burn off excess fat.

We all have a basic 'resting' heart rate (our heart rate when we're at our most relaxed) and a 'maximum' heart rate. Most people's maximum heart rate will be about 220 minus their age. So if you're 35 years old and new to exercise, your maximum heart rate will be around 185 beats per minute. You can practise taking your pulse by counting the number of beats in 15 seconds, then multiplying by 4 to reach a figure for 'beats per minute'.

- *To find your maximum heart rate, subtract your age from 220.*
- *A low target rate during exercise will be 50 per cent of your maximum.*
- *A high target heart rate during exercise will be 85 per cent of your maximum.*

While this formula incorporates your age, it does not incorporate your fitness level, so beginners should work at the low end. Only competing athletes should aim for the high end.

To get the best fitness results, it's recommended that you vary the intensity of your workouts, with shorter spells at your high heart rate and longer spells at your low heart rate. Your body actually responds differently to these two types of exercise and to achieve rounded fitness you'll want to include both types.

An aerobic exercise is one in which you work out consistently for 20–60 minutes within your THR (Target Heart Rate) range. I recommend that you do this at least three times a week.

In time you'll know what your 'right' target feels like and you won't have to bother taking your pulse. But for beginners, you should check your pulse periodically throughout your workout. This method is an accurate way to maintain a pace that's not only safe but which also builds aerobic capacity and burns fat.

How Can I Tell If I Am Overdoing It?

You'll know if you're overdoing it if your chest starts pounding like crazy or if you feel dizzy or faint. Just cool down for about 5–10 minutes before ending your workout. If this keeps up and you're working below your high rate, see a doctor.

If all the maths and pulse-taking is too much for you, I really recommend you buy an *Electronic Heart Rate Monitor*. These handy little gadgets provide an instant read-out of your heart rate as you exercise. Prices start from around £30.

4. YOUR FIRST STEPS 10-MINUTE WORKOUT

This First Steps Workout is an ideal all-round aerobic routine which can be used by anyone from total beginners to the more advanced. As well as being a good routine for increasing aerobic capacity and toning your heart and cardiovascular system, it also incorporates moves that will tone and sculpt.

You'll need a skipping rope and a pair of 5 to 15 lb weights (a couple of half-litre bottles of water or tins of beans will do). For all of the following jumping and jogging moves, make sure you're on a shock-absorbing surface. Avoid concrete floors or pavements; instead, jump on a gym mat, on a springy wood floor or on the ground – an earth or sand track, a sandy beach or a firm lawn will do.

23

FIGURE-EIGHT ROPE SWINGS

Beginners   1–3 minutes
Intermediate/advanced   2–4 minutes

A   Stand with your hands together, holding a skipping rope at waist height.

B   Keeping your legs slightly bent and shoulder-width apart, tuck your elbows into your sides and swing the rope in figure eights in front of you. Keep the rope movements small, turning it from your wrists and forearms rather than your shoulders.

C   As you swing, jump, feet together, from side to side. Do not jump over the rope; swing it in front of your body. Keep your body weight on the balls of your feet, but make sure your whole foot lands after each jump. To minimize impact, stay low to the ground. Vary the intensity by moderating the speed of your jumps.

TRIPLE BICEPS CURL

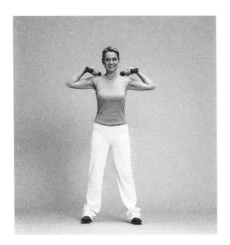

Beginners	15–20 reps
Intermediate/advanced	25–30 reps

A   Stand with feet hip-width apart, weights in both hands, arms extended straight out to the sides, palms facing upward. Hold your arms away from your rib cage, elbows 4 to 6 inches (10–15 cm) from your ribs.

B   Curl the weights into your shoulders by bending your elbows, then straighten your arms back out, away from your rib cage.

C   Move your (straightened) arms closer together so that they point out at 45° angles, then perform one biceps curl with both arms.

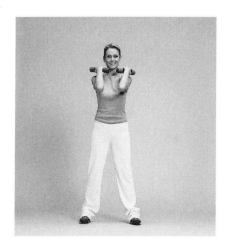

D   Move your arms, extended below shoulder level, in front of your body, and curl the weights in towards your chin. Straighten your elbows. Reverse sequence. Repeat.

AB PUNCH CRUNCH

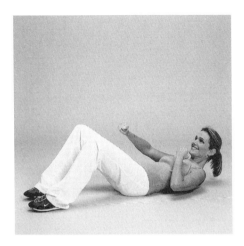

Beginners   15–20 reps
Intermediate/advanced   25–30 reps

A   Lie back, knees bent and feet flat. Crunch up as high as you can. This
    means pulling your abdomen in and up to lift your shoulders and rib
    cage off the floor, keeping your shoulders back and relaxed.
B   Alternate four quick straight punches right through your legs. Throw
    four more punches on the way back down – this counts as one rep.
    Crunch through the full range of motion with your abs tight.

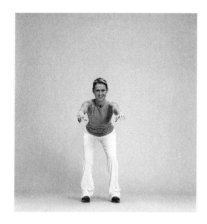

| Beginners | 2–5 reps |
| Intermediate/advanced | 3–8 reps |

28

A   Start in a semi-squat position, knees bent, hands above thighs.

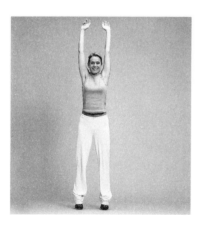

B   Spring up and reach arms overhead to jump as high as you can. Land softly. March in place to rest for 15 seconds, then jump again.

Fight Fat, Fight Fatigue

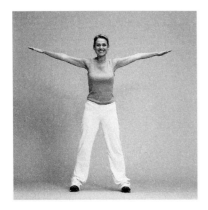

Beginners   1 minute
Intermediate/advanced   1–2 minutes

A   Starting with feet together, jump out so your feet are shoulder-width apart. Lift arms out in a 'T' position.

B   Jump back; drop arms by sides.

C   Jump forward and raise straight arms in front to shoulder level.

29

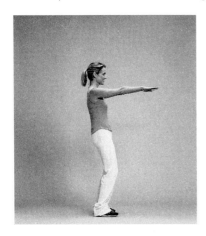

D   Jump back, dropping arms to thighs.

First Steps to a New You

THE JUMP-UP JACK

This is the basic jump-up jack, a perfect anaerobic exercise that has stood the test of time. Growing up, you did them in the gym. Then in aerobics classes, they appeared again. Even professional athletes include this classic exercise in their training regimes because it is so effective. This seemingly simple move has endured the test of time because it uses and conditions so many muscles at once. The jumping jack also can help raise your body temperature at the end of a warm-up or increase exercise intensity in a cardio workout. Perhaps the best thing about it is that you don't need any equipment at all – your body provides all the resistance you need. By jumping higher and more force-fully, you can strengthen and tone your buttocks and legs, while improving your ability to jump.

Since this is a high-impact move, be sure to attempt it only at the end of your warm-up or during the cardio portion of your regular exercise programme. Also, wear appropriate workout shoes and perform the move on a soft surface such as grass, sand or a cushioned floor (avoid cement surfaces) to protect your joints.

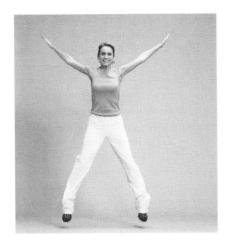

A   Stand with your feet facing forward, slightly apart, hands by your sides. Bend your knees slightly and then, pushing down with your feet, jump high into the air, bringing your legs and arms out to the sides, arms at shoulder height. As you land, your feet should hit the ground slightly more than hip-width apart. Upon landing, also bend slightly at the ankles, knees and hips so that the landing is smooth and soft.

B   Reverse the move, this time jumping your legs back together and bringing your arms back down to your sides to return to starting position.

Remember: *Throughout the exercise, focus on keeping your abs tight and your torso in line with your pelvis. Avoid leaning forward during the preparation phase and jerking backward on the takeoff. Also, try to keep the middle of your kneecaps over the second toes when your knees bend during the preparation and the landing. Be careful not to allow your knees to fall inward relative to your feet (a common mistake). As your strength and form improve, focus on jumping up even higher, while maintaining good placement of the knees and spine.*

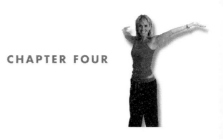

CHAPTER FOUR

STRETCHING

S tretching is as important to your overall fitness as weight-training and aerobics. Whether you're as active as a dancer, avid exerciser or simply interested in optimal well-being, stretching should be a regular part of your programme. The benefits go beyond simply increasing flexibility.

33

- *Stretching can make you feel more relaxed by reducing muscle tension. It can also prevent muscle strains, promote circulation and prevent and even cure certain types of back pain.*

It always amazes me, when I am at the gym, how many people I see jump straight onto the treadmill, bike or rower and go hell for leather. Then they can't understand why they have pulled or strained a muscle. Warming up and stretching before and after any exercise or sport is probably the most important part of a session and yet is probably the most neglected. Stretching is vital, as it allows greater flexibility and avoids damaging the muscles that you are working.

Stretch for at least 5 minutes before and after working each individual muscle group.

If you weight-train or get a vigorous workout, stretching will help your muscles stay lithe and limber – and there is some truth that stretching can help make a muscle appear longer and smoother.

Warning: Although stretching is one of the safest types of exercise, *there are a few conditions where you shouldn't stretch.* Unless a physician or other competent medical provider says otherwise, you shouldn't stretch the muscles around a bone that's been recently fractured, or an area that has been recently sprained or strained, especially the muscles of the back of the neck. Of course, if you have a question about the safety aspects of a specific stretch or stretching in general, you should consult a professional.

Important: If you are not stretching immediately after your workout, you will need to perform a warm-up prior to stretching. *Never stretch cold.* Try 5 to 10 minutes of low-intensity aerobic activity, such as light running on the spot, to get your heart rate up.

TIPS

1   *Always warm up before stretching.*
2   *Always hold your stretch for 10–30 seconds. Never bounce during a stretch.*
3   *Do not hold your breath while stretching.*
4   *You should feel a tightness, but never pain. Do not force a joint and do not extend it beyond its normal range of motion.*
5   *Perform each stretch at least twice.*
6   *Stretch slowly: ease in and out of every stretch slowly and smoothly.*

YOUR STRETCHING PROGRAMME

ANKLES

A   Sit on the floor with one leg extended. Lift the other leg, knee bent.

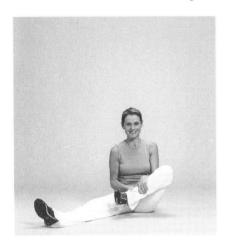

B   Rotate your ankles in several directions while providing slight resist-
     ance with your hand.

LOWER BACK

A   Lie on your back, making sure your lower back is flat on the floor.

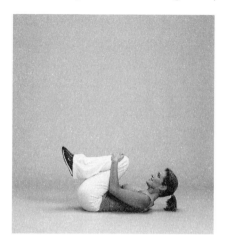

B   Pull your knees to your chest.

NECK

A   Bend your neck towards your right shoulder, then down, then finally towards your left shoulder.

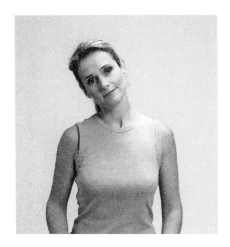

B   Stop at each position for at least 8 seconds.

37

Stretching

UPPER BODY

A   Your feet should be shoulder-width apart. Keep your knees slightly bent and bend to the side at your waist.

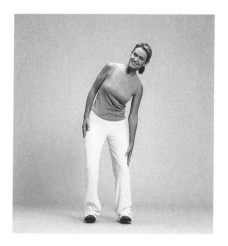

38

BACK

A   Lie on your back, one leg extended. Bring the other leg across your body with your knee bent. Turn your head in the opposite direction.

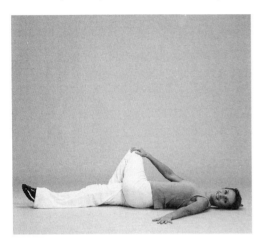

B   To increase the stretch, place your hand on your bent knee.

Stretching

SHOULDERS AND CHEST

A   Clasp your hands behind your back. Lift your arms up slowly until you feel the stretch.

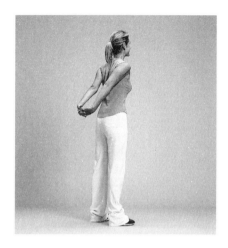

QUADRICEPS

A   Hold your leg with the opposite arm. Do not lock the knee joint of your straight leg.

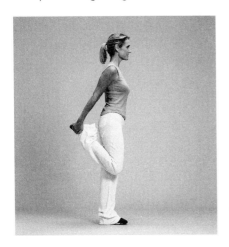

B   This exercise can also be done lying on your stomach.

HAMSTRINGS

A   Sit on the floor, one leg extended. Place one foot against the thigh of the extended leg. Bend forward from the hip. Do not bend your neck down.

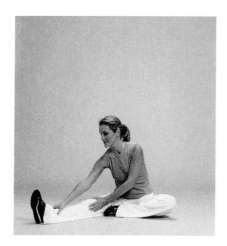

CALVES

A   Place one leg extended behind you, heels flat on the floor. Place your body weight on your front leg, with your knees bent. Keep your hips forward.

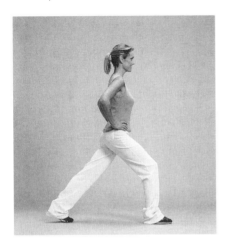

TRICEPS AND SHOULDERS

Gently pull your elbow behind your head.

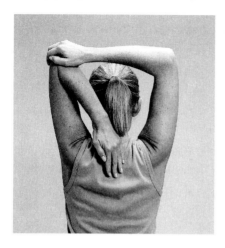

MORE STRETCHING EXERCISES

I have included additional quad and hamstring stretches, since these are areas of the body which get a lot of stress in activities such as running and are often injured by not enough preparation.

Additional Quad Stretch

Stretches the front muscles of the thigh – the quadriceps

Workout Prescription   After each action, switch legs.
                                 Work for 5 minutes.

STARTING POSITION

You may need to hold on to something such as the back of a chair to maintain your balance. Stand upright on your right leg with that knee slightly bent.

1   Grasp your left foot around the ankle and slowly move your heel towards your buttocks, keeping your knees together. Hold this position for about 10 seconds, making sure your back is straight and your stomach is tucked in.
2   During this time, contract your buttock muscles, drawing them downward to increase the stretch on the front of the leg.
3   Change legs and repeat.

Tip

To prevent over-stretching or injury, try not to let your back arch, and keep your left knee pointing directly downwards, so as to keep your bones and muscles in the correct aligned position.

Additional Hamstring Stretch

Stretches rear thigh, calves and lower back

Workout Prescription | Try 5 reps, holding for 30–60 seconds.

STARTING POSITION

Place your straight right leg on a chair or bench, foot flexed, with our left knee unlocked and left foot on the floor.

1   Slowly rounding your back forward, bring your chest towards your right knee, placing both hands just above your right knee to hold.
2   Breathe deeply, keeping your neck in line with your upper back.
3   Switch sides and repeat.

Tip

After you've mastered the basic stretch, try bringing your chest as close as you comfortably can to your right knee, placing both hands under your right calf to hold.

Additional Calf Stretch

One of the most common tennis injuries is calf strain, so I cannot over-emphasize the importance of warming up and stretching before any sport or exercise. The more flexible the muscle, the more efficient it becomes. Stretching may not be the most fun you've ever had, and if you are like me you'd rather clean the car or do the ironing, but miss stretching out and you may wish you hadn't. This calf stretch is easy and can be done at any time.

Workout Prescription   Hold for 10 seconds then change legs and repeat on the other side.

STARTING POSITION
Using the wall or a chair as support, place one foot behind the other.

1   With your front knee slightly bent, back knee straight and heel down, lean your hips forward, stretching your back leg while really feeling the stretch in the calf muscle.
2   Hold for 10 seconds, then change legs and repeat on the other side.

Tip
Make sure the toes of both your feet are facing forwards.

THE BALANCE-OUT-YOUR-BODY STRETCH

Do you tend to favour your left side over your right side or vice versa? Do you have muscle strain along one side of your body or lower back? This soothing side-stretch will help to redress the balance.

You may think of yourself as right-handed or left-handed, but chances are you also emphasize one side of your body without even realizing it. Have you ever watched two women gossip? Watch how they shift their weight onto one hip. When you hold a toddler, which hip do you favour? Even just standing up, most people tend to shift their weight onto one leg, or if you participate in a lateral sport like golf or tennis or bowling, you're probably emphasizing one side over another. Over time this can lead to muscle strain along one side of your body, as well as lower back pain. This is a fairly common problem that tends to build up slowly and then reach a point where you're in pain. But that doesn't mean you have to live with it. This pose is great for alleviating back or side strain, or simply for giving yourself a soothing side, bottom and lower-back stretch.

To Get into Position

1 Cross your left leg over your right. Raise your right arm over your head, left arm to the side, parallel to the floor.
2 Look over your left arm and breathe deeply as you hold the position for 5 seconds.

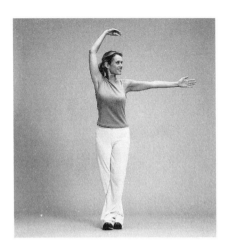

3   If you want to increase the side stretch, bend slightly to your left. Now switch sides, with your right leg over your left.

But you're not off the hook yet! When you're walking, standing or sitting as you go about your day, pay attention. You may be favouring one leg over the other. Focus on centring your weight and using both sides of your body – and you'll be on the way to feeling more balanced.

Tips

1   **Breathe right:** *Inhale slowly and exhale deeply in order to relax further into the stretch.*
2   **Elongate your arm:** *Try to extend your left arm as far away from your body as it can go.*
3   **Lengthen your spine:** *Lift your upper body away from your hips.*
4   **Lower your hip:** *Push right down and away from the body.*
5   **Bend your knees:** *If this stretch bothers your knees at all, bend them slightly.*

Stretching

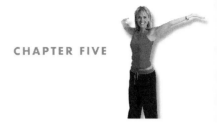

CHAPTER FIVE

HOW TO BE A GOOD SPORT

Regular everyday activities such as tennis, swimming, running and cycling can be hugely fun ways to burn off the calories and tone up those muscles. If you make a little bit of sporting fun part of your all-round exercise programme, you will notice the benefits faster. What's more, this sort of exercise gets you out of the house and makes you happy. You already knew this, but now it's official: research shows that a good workout beats the blues.

51

For years I've called my running shoes my 'soul' prescription. On the days when I feel sad or overwhelmed, when I argue with a friend or miss someone close or wonder what's going on, I head out for a run. Experts have concluded that exercise is a powerful way to defeat depression, release stress and set off an explosion of mood-boosting chemicals in your brain. If you're stuck in a low mood, you can significantly improve your state of mind in the long term by doing a low or moderate intensity work-out for 20–60 minutes at least 3 times a week for a minimum of 5 weeks.

Whether that exercise is aerobic (walking or running) or non-aerobic (strength-training) doesn't make a difference. The bottom line: Get your butt off the couch and exercise and you will boost your health and your mood.

And here's more good news:

YOU BURN OFF STRESS

Working out is one of the few ways we can give ourselves a 'time-out' from job pressures and family demands. Even quiet activities like yoga or stretching can grant you the space you need to rejuvenate.

WORKING OUT BOOSTS YOUR BRAIN'S 'HAPPY' CHEMICALS

Similar to antidepressant drugs, exercise appears to cause brain neuro-transmitters to up levels of endorphins called serotonin and norepi-nephrine, which are thought to boost mood.

YOU BANISH THE BODY BLUES

Even if you don't shed a pound through your workouts, exercise improves the way you feel about yourself, both inside and out. Building up from a walking routine to running a 10K, for instance, helps you appreciate the strength, power and performance your body has to offer.

CREATING A FEEL-GREAT WORKOUT

You don't have to run yourself ragged to shake a case of the blues, just about any type of exercise can work. The key: Exercise consistently. The American College of Sports and Medicine recommends exercising 3–5 days a week for 20–60 minutes at 55–80 per cent of your maximum heart rate. Round out your weekly routine with 2 or 3 sessions each of strength-training and stretching. It's OK to combine your activities. For example, one day you might walk for 20 minutes, work your lower body with squats or lunges, then cool down by stretching the major muscle groups. Mix and match from my recommended activities below to find a well-balanced formula for your own happiness.

Three to Five Days a Week

Try:

CARDIO

Mood-boosting secret

When you raise your heart rate, your brain increases its secretion of feel-good endorphins.

20–60 minutes of:

- cycling
- running
- in-line skating
- swimming
- aerobic dance or workout video

Two to Three Days a Week

Try:

STRENGTH-TRAINING

Mood-boosting secret

Studies have shown that aerobic and strength-training exercises are equally effective in reducing depression.

1–3 sets of 8–10 reps of:

- lunges or squats
- abdominal crunches
- press-ups or bench-presses
- arm lift and curls (with 3, 5 or 8 lb weights)

Two to Three Days a Week

Try:

FLEXIBILITY

Mood-boosting secret   Just having a good time out from daily pressures can reduce anxiety.

A quiet session of:

- yoga
- Pilates
- stretching the major muscle groups, holding each for 10–30 seconds
  - lower body: fronts of thighs, backs of thighs, buttocks and calves
  - upper body: abdominals, front of arms, backs of arms, upper back, lower back, shoulders and neck

One or Two Days a Week

Try:

ACTIVE SOCIALIZING

Mood-boosting secret   Contact with 'life-reinforcers' (family, friends) keeps you from feeling sad or isolated.

Fight Fat, Fight Fatigue

A few examples:

- playing with the kids in the park
- window-shopping with a friend
- a pick-up game of volleyball or tennis
- bowling with co-workers
- walking the dog

MY GET-REAL GUIDE FOR PAIN-FREE,

PERMANENT WEIGHTLOSS

Walking

It doesn't matter where you walk, just stride out at a brisk pace for 20–30 minutes, preferably 3 times a week, and you will notice an improvement in your fitness level in no time at all. You could even take your trainers to work and spend half your lunch-hour walking.

Throwing yourself too enthusiastically into an exercise regime you're not yet fit enough or mentally prepared for is the quickest way to lose interest. If you are unfit and new to exercise, start off with walking. You don't need any equipment, money or even that much time. Walking can lead to motivation, enthusiasm and the exercising habit.

Here's my get-real guide for pain-free, permanent weight loss:

1 Always start with 5 minutes of gentle walking followed by some light stretching as your warm-up.
2 Concentrate on maintaining a good posture by keeping your shoulders back and your rib cage lifted.

3   Strike forward with your heel and push off with your back foot. Gradually increase the length and speed of your stride, but never over-stretch. Pull your abdominals in and 'think tall'. Look forward, not down.

THREE WAYS TO WALK HARDER

1   Carry light handweights, half-litre bottles of water or tins of beans so you can exercise your upper body while you walk.
2   For increased intensity and more variety, try interval training. Walk at a fast pace for, say, 400 m. Then slow down for the next 200 m. Repeat as many times as is comfortable.
3   Add hill-walking to your programme for a real challenge.

Tip

Listen to your body: Increase the level when you no longer feel challenged; reduce the level when you feel tired. If you feel slightly breathless but comfortable, you are walking at the right level. At the end of your walk, always slow down gradually and repeat your stretching routine.

Speedwalking

About 4 miles per hour.
This is my number-one aerobics choice. Speedwalking is ideal for novices. Just lace up and walk quickly, swinging your arms. While the waddle-like walk may look more like Donald Duck at times, this exercise is no quack! It's safe, easy and something you can do anywhere, anytime. It's also perfect for those who can't afford gyms or wouldn't be caught dead in one. I recommend working out with a friend. Mine is Hugo, my bearded collie, who keeps my pulse up there. Teaming up not only keeps you from dropping out, but will give you a motivational soulmate who can share your accomplishments.

For those of you who prefer solitude, speedwalking lets you walk away from it all (your job, boss, boyfriend, the kids) and return in 30 minutes feeling like a new woman. Walk to your favourite music, that's what I always do. The faster the beat, the faster you walk.

Running

You can set your own pace, go where you like, it's cheap – and it's a great way to stay in shape. It's a huge calorie burner – expect to use up 600–800 calories an hour, depending on your body weight and how fast you run.

Running gives your heart and lungs a great workout and it also tones up your legs and bottom. If you keep going long enough – usually about half an hour – you may also experience a 'runner's high', an exhilarating state caused by endorphins (the body's natural painkillers).

If you haven't run further than to the bus stop since you were a child, taking up a running programme can seem daunting. A common mistake is starting off too fast, so that you soon get out of breath and can't continue. Instead, begin by walking and then gradually introduce short sections of slow running. Return to walking when you start to tire. You should feel warm and glowing, but not so out of breath you can't carry on a conversation. Try and go out for between 20 and 30 minutes, and keep alternating walking and running until you're doing more running than walking. It won't be long before you can run continuously for 30 minutes.

TAKE IT EASY

- If you're already fit but not used to running, go carefully at first.
- Warm up by walking at a moderate pace for a few minutes.
- Taper down at end of a run by walking.
- Do some simple stretches after your warm-up and at end of the walk, concentrating on the calves, thighs, hip flexors and hamstrings.

How to Be a Good Sport

PROGRESS

Once you can run non-stop for about 30 minutes, start adding variety and challenges by incorporating the following elements into your training regimen:

LONG, SLOW DISTANCE

Running at a pace that's slow enough to maintain for half an hour or more.

Keep the intensity low and don't start off too fast. For beginners, a fraction quicker than a brisk walk is fast enough. This method burns fat and is good for weight loss. It should form the basis of your training.

CONTINUOUS FAST RUNNING

Running fast so you feel you are working hard.

At first you won't be able to keep going for long at this intensity, probably only 5 minutes, but it boosts fitness, your heart beats faster and your body has to transport oxygen more quickly.

HILLS

Running uphill increases your heart rate and improves aerobic fitness.

Hill-running is also good for your running style, as it requires a more vigorous arm action and a higher knee lift, which will also strengthen your legs. Start by warming up on the flat for 5–10 minutes, then run hard up a small hill and back down the other side. Let yourself recover with some gentle walking for the same amount of time as it took you to get up and down the hill. Repeat this pattern 3–4 times, as it really is a good way to boost your fitness and stop you from getting bored.

INTERVAL TRAINING

Alternating between running and recovery for a set time.

Intensity and duration depend on factors such as fitness levels and ability. You may run fast for 30 seconds, then walk briskly or run slowly for one minute to recover before repeating the pattern. Eventually you should do more running than recovering. It will improve speed, endurance and oxygen transport, as well as condition your muscles for fast running.

STAIRS

Doing stairs will increase your power and stamina and give your legs a killer workout.

A good sturdy set of stairs is a necessity. Begin with a mile warm-up and do single and doubles (two steps at a time). You can run up, jog over, jog or walk down and so on. Or do singles all the way up and doubles on the way back. At the end, cool down with a slow jog for a couple of minutes and stretch out. Stop when you get tired or notice your form begin to slip.

Tips

Choose shoes that have been bio-mechanically designed with running in mind. Cross-training shoes are meant to be used for very short distances only, when running is just one of many activities that you are doing on a regular basis. To keep motivated, find a friend to join you, preferably of the same sex and similar standard or you may be put off by not being able to keep up. For full details of events and race diaries telephone Runner's World on 0800 731 0622.

Cycling

Cycling firms your bottom, tones your thighs, burns fat, reduces stress and boosts your energy. It's an excellent form of aerobic exercise.

HOW TO GET STARTED

To improve your cardiovascular fitness, you need to cycle continuously for 20 minutes or more 3–4 times a week. Always remember to stretch, warm up, cool down and stretch again. The proper cycling action is a complete circle, pushing down for the first half of the stroke and pulling up with the second, using every muscle in your legs.

USING A STATIONARY BIKE

Depending on your fitness level, try to incorporate 10-second bursts of higher intensity training, gradually building up to intervals of 30–60 seconds or more. While it boosts your training level, it also prevents boredom.

FOR THE ADVANCED ONLY

After cycling at your normal mph for 5 minutes, jump-start your pedalling pace for 20–30 seconds, then drop back to your regular speed for another 5 minutes. Repeat these bursts throughout your routine – I promise you'll see a difference in stamina and body shape within a month.

Tip

It's important to adjust the saddle height to suit you. When sitting on the bike, your knee should be slightly bent on the down stroke. Always carry water and a banana or energy-boosting cereal bar.

Tennis

Calories burned per half hour: 175 in doubles; 225 in singles.

It's never too late for anyone to start – and with the number of calories it burns and the muscles brought into play, tennis is an ideal aerobic sport. It takes advantage of hand-eye co-ordination, explosive speed and quick changes of direction, all of which help burn fat and challenge your mind.

Try this: Tennis can be played at any public tennis court, either for free or for a small fee, or at most schools or colleges after hours. To improve your game, try taking a couple of lessons. A half-hour private, one-on-one lesson costs under £10, depending on where you live. You can also look into classes, whether you're a beginner, intermediate or advanced player, as they are normally divided into groups according to ability and are sponsored by local parks and leisure clubs.

Tip
If you are a newcomer to this game, always remember to wear comfortable clothing and that you'll need a good pair of supportive tennis shoes.

Boxercise

A 4-minute routine to break you out into a sweat.

Time management is crucial for today's busy, fitness-conscious woman. Squeezing in a workout during a hectic day is always a challenge, so with that in mind, this 4-minute boxercise routine can be done at home, in a hotel room or even at work.

STARTING POSITION
Start by using a diagonal stance and lift and lower your front knee. Then pivot your torso and punch with your back arm, keeping your thumbs on the outside of your fist. Do a set of 4 punches and then incorporate 8 jumping jacks to transition you to the other side. Then repeat. 4 minutes in total.

JUMPING JACKS
Everyone knows how to do a jumping jack *(see page 30)*, but my main tip is to tell you to concentrate on pulling your arms into your body as you close the jack.

Keep your abs in and shoulders down when you punch.

Skipping

A speedy cardiovascular shape-up.

Skipping is so easy to learn and the only equipment you need is a rope and a pair of supportive shoes. You can do it almost anywhere, at any time, so I suggest everybody buys everybody else a skipping rope as a Christmas or birthday present. It provides a great cardiovascular shape-up in a relatively short time. This is also an exercise the whole family can do. Have competitions, see who can skip the longest or count how many skips you can do in a set time. It's also a great calorie-burner and it's fun.

Tip

Use your wrists and forearms to turn the rope; don't turn from the shoulders. Remember your feet, too – don't jump on your toes, and let your heels help absorb the impact. Keep your knees bent slightly; your knees may not be taking a beating, but your feet and calves should be. Remember, if you've led a relatively sedentary life for some time, get your doctor's permission before skipping.

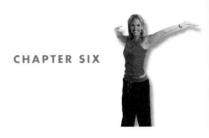

CHAPTER SIX

WORKING YOUR UPPER BODY

Your upper body includes your arms, shoulders, back and cleavage. Many women are not naturally 'strong' in the upper body and often it's a neglected area – so if saggy arms, chubby shoulders or a fat back are something you're looking to avoid, read on! You'll be happy to hear that this is one area of the body that responds quickly to a little effort in the right direction and with the right diet plus regular use of some of the following resistance exercises you can:

- Lift and strengthen your chest – providing definition in the cleavage area.
- Sculpt and define your arms – minimizing upper arm 'batwings'.
- Tone your shoulders – to achieve a firm, distinctive line.
- Strengthen your back – gain elegance that you'll want to show off and say goodbye to many nagging aches.

63

The exercises that follow are carefully chosen to work, tone and strengthen precisely the right individual muscle groups to produce the shape you want. You should select at least 2 exercises from this upper body chapter, and perform them 3 times per week.

Remember:

1 *Don't work the same muscle groups two days in a row – without adequate recovery time you won't get the benefits and you might simply end up injured. So – pace yourself!*
2 *Always be sure to warm up before you start and to cool down and stretch each time you work out.*

64

THE CHEST

Firm your pectorals and sculpt a sexy upper body

Chest exercises are the same for both men and women. However, I am aiming my comments at women in this section, since women have a bosom, which looks all the better for a boost. By following these exercises you will give your body an experience that will uplift your spirits and your bust line at the same time. Developing your pectoral muscles will help support the breast tissue, which will give your breasts a fuller, more rounded and youthful appearance and, as a bonus, you'll get a little extra cleavage for those sexy plunging necklines, bustiers and strappy little dresses.

The first exercise, my simple knee press-up, is guaranteed to do the job because it zeros in on 'cleavage central' – the upper and inner area of the pectoral muscles. You'll find that not only does it ward off the effects of gravity, but it will also improve your posture.

The Simple Knee Press-up

Tones the chest, back of the arms, shoulders and stomach muscles

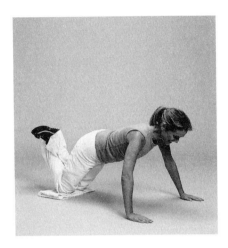

Workout Prescription | 3 sets of 12–15 repetitions, breaking for 30–40 seconds between sets.

STARTING POSITION

Kneeling on the floor, place your hands right below your shoulders. Your knees should be a few inches behind your hips, back straight. Look at the floor to keep your neck in alignment with your spine.

1   Inhale, then exhale and slowly lower your upper body down towards the floor until your shoulders come into line with your elbows.

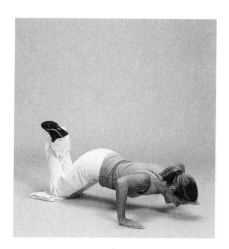

2   Hold this position for the count of 3, then inhale and slowly raise your body to the starting position, using your stomach muscles.

Tip

For even faster results you can do press-ups the hard way – on your toes, with straight legs. Make sure that you do not lock your elbows.

Fight Fat, Fight Fatigue

Bust-booster

Next is a bust-booster that's a little more advanced. You need a bench press and a barbell (any kind of bar or broom handle will work as well, as long as it's not too heavy). This exercise strengthens the triceps, front shoulders and chest.

RECOMMENDED RESISTANCE
- Beginners: 2–4 lb
- Intermediates: 5–8 lb
- Advanced: 8–10 lb

Workout Prescription   8–12 repetitions, repeating 2–3 times with a 30 to 40-second rest in between.

STARTING POSITION

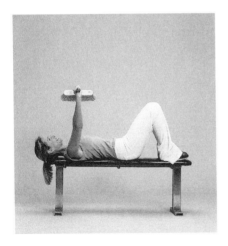

Lie on a flat bench with your knees bent and feet flat on the edge of the bench. Hold a barbell (or bar or broom handle) above your chest with an overhand grip, hands slightly wider than shoulder-width apart, keeping your abdomen contracted and a slight natural arch in your back.

1 Keeping your back and shoulders on the bench, inhale as you lower the bar towards your chest until your elbows are even with your shoulders.

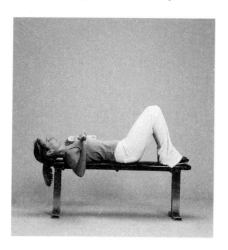

2 Exhale and press back up to starting position and repeat, concentrating on contracting your chest muscles at the top of the movement.

Tip

If you are using an adjustable gym bench, you can add these additional variations to your workout:

1 For your upper chest, set the bench at a 45° incline and lie with your head at the highest point and your feet flat on the floor.
2 For your lower chest, lie with your head at the lowest point of the bench and your feet flat on the floor.

THE BACK

A strong back will:

- improve your posture
- balance your strength between front and back and upper and lower body
- help to eliminate lower back pain by strengthening muscles along the spine
- increase upper-body width, giving the appearance of a smaller waist
- eliminate back flabbiness and overhanging fat

The perfect physique begins with a strong back, but it is an area that is commonly neglected, perhaps because you can't see it. Every day, without knowing it, many of us are creating a strength imbalance in our upper body. Whether driving, lifting or typing away on the keyboard, you're positioning your arms in front of you so your back gets forgotten, and often you slouch. This is why back strain is one of the most common reasons for people being off work. On another level, a flabby back with love handles and bulges over the top of your bra, bikini top or that pretty backless slinky gown isn't very attractive and, as many movie stars have recently discovered, that plunging backless look is every bit as sexy as the perfect cleavage. So do yourself a favour. Make a special effort to remember your back, because even if you can't see it, it will be worth it.

69

THE UPPER BACK – TRAP TRAINING

Ignoring the trapezius – the upper back – is a big mistake, considering that it takes up nearly the same surface area as the stomach region many people pay so much attention to. Toned traps look good and they also play a key role in almost any sport. Whenever you raise your arms overhead, for example, your traps help lift your shoulder blades, which allows you to complete that bowl or tennis serve. The muscle becomes more important in football, cricket, diving and other activities in which head and neck absorb impact. It is also mainly responsible for giving you that 'burn' when you walk through an airport lugging a pair of heavy suitcases and bearing the brunt of the punishment when you struggle to open a heavy door.

Lat Pullover

Strengthens middle back and shoulders

Workout Prescription

10–12 reps. Rest for 30 seconds. Repeat 2–3 times.

STARTING POSITION

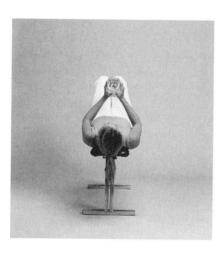

Lie on your back on a bench with your feet flat on the bench or the floor and your head at the other end.

1   With both hands, hold one end of a dumbbell (a half-litre bottle of water or tin of beans will do) over your chest with arms slightly bent.

2   Inhale and move the dumbbell through an arc-like pattern over your head and slightly behind you.

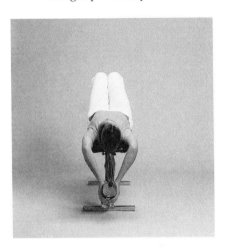

3   Exhale and lift the dumbbell slowly back over your chest and repeat.

Tip

Count slowly to 4 on the lift and to 4 again while exhaling, returning once again to the starting position. Be sure to move through your full range of motion.

Working your Upper Body

The Back Extension with a Twist

Tones and strengthens your lower and upper back

Workout Prescription   3 sets of 8–12 reps.

STARTING POSITION

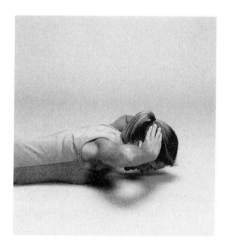

Lie stomach-down on the floor and place your hands either against your forehead or on the back of your head, elbows out to the sides.

1 Contract your stomach and buttock muscles hard and slowly lift your right shoulder and chest off the floor (keep your left elbow on the floor).
2 Twist up and back through the right side of your torso until your right elbow points up to the ceiling.

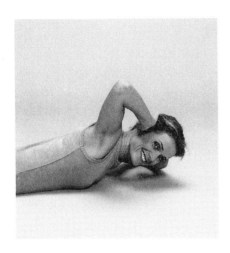

3   Keep your head perfectly still and your chin down to avoid straining your neck. Hold this position for 5 seconds, then slowly switch sides.

Tip

Make sure you keep your hipbones on the floor at all times and flex your buttock muscles as you raise and lower yourself.

SHOULDERS

Toned shoulders will define your silhouette and help to keep your posture upright so you stand straighter, look younger and feel elegant. Shoulder exercises will also get rid of 'keyboard stoop' and ensure you don't develop a 'hunch'.

Press to De-stress

Tones, strengthens and relaxes all those tight shoulder muscles
This exercise is a fast stress-buster and will help you to both stand straighter and look younger.

Workout prescription

Warm up with 15 minutes of brisk walking or light jogging. Start with 10 reps. Build up to 20 reps. One set.

STARTING POSITION

Sit tall at the edge of a bench, feet together and flat on the floor. Hold a light dumbbell in each hand (this can be half-litre bottles of water or tins of beans), arms at your sides with your palms facing your thighs.

1   Slowly exhale and lift the weights out to your sides until your arms are parallel to the floor. Inhale and lower the weights back to your sides. Do 10 reps.

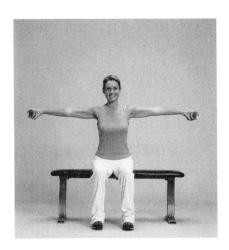

2   Exhale and raise both arms straight in front of you, parallel to the floor.
Inhale and lower your arms. Repeat 10 times.

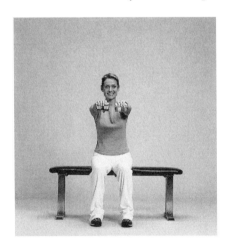

3 Lean forward at your waist so that your back is almost parallel to the floor. Your arms should be hanging straight down. Slowly, exhale and raise the weights up and out to the sides until they are parallel to the floor. Inhale and lower. Repeat 10 times.

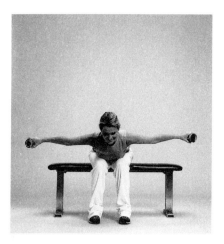

4 Repeat this whole exercise twice more, building up to 20 reps each time.

Tip
Make sure you keep your tummy muscles tight at all times.

The Dumbbell Lateral Raise

Tones and strengthens the shoulder muscles

Workout Prescription   12–15 reps. Repeat 3 times.

Also known as the 'Big Lift', this is a way to delay physical ageing without risk or dramatic expense. This method can work whether you're aged 18 or 90, fit or unfit, hoping to build bone density, lose fat and gain strength and energy, or wanting nothing more than to look better in a sleeveless T-shirt and never having to wear shoulder pads again. It can be done at home or at work. It will make you stronger and build muscles, which means you will be burning more calories even when sleeping. Its benefits become visible in just a few weeks, so stick at it!

STARTING POSITION

Sit on the edge of a bench or chair with your back straight and shoulders relaxed. Your feet should be flat on the floor, shoulder-width apart. Hold a dumbbell (half-litre bottle of water or tin of beans) in each hand with your hands in front of you and bend your arms at a 90° angle so that your palms are facing each other.

1   Inhale. Slowly raise your weights out to your sides to shoulder level or slightly higher, leading the movement with your knuckles and keeping the angle at your elbow joint 'fixed'. Keep your back and shoulders relaxed but fixed throughout. Try and maintain the 90° bend at the elbows throughout the movement.

2 Exhale. Lower the dumbbells under control to the starting position.

Tip

The dumbbells should be slightly rotated as they are raised (i.e. the thumbs face downward) so that at the finish position, shoulder height or marginally above, the dumbbells are parallel to the floor, palms facing down.

The Upright Row

Tones the deltoids (shoulder muscles), trapezius (upper back) and biceps (upper arms)

Workout Prescription

12–15 reps. Repeat 3 times. Use an exercise bar. (You can buy one, but any bar will do – such as a broom or mop handle.)

This is a fantastic exercise specially designed to help define your shoulders, upper back and biceps, enabling you to wear any of those sleeveless or strapless outfits that show off a great tan. And you'll gain the benefits of looking and feeling on top of the world.

STARTING POSITION

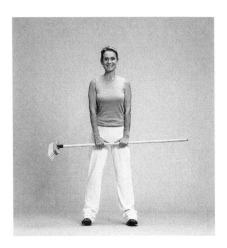

Stand upright, feet shoulder-width apart. Hold the bar so that it is resting at the top of your thighs, arms straight. Grip the bar with your palms facing your body, leaving 3 to 4 inches (7.5–10 cm) between your hands.

1   Inhale, lift your chest and tighten your abdominal muscles.

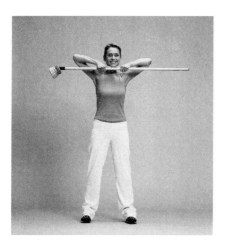

2   Exhale and slowly lift the bar up under your chin, keeping your elbows pointed out and up. Make sure your back is locked and your upper back is stationary at all times, then slowly lower the bar and return to the starting position.

Tip

Try not to swing or arch your back when you begin to feel tired. Keep your elbows higher than your chin at all times.

Fight Fat, Fight Fatigue

ARMS

Muscle groups: Biceps (front of arms)
                                       Triceps (back of arms)

Don't think that only weight-lifters need strong arms. Arms are often the first areas to go on a woman and show her age. I call saggy underarms 'batwings' – and who needs those? There is no doubt that nicely toned, shapely arms are feminine and means you don't have to cover up all those pretty sleeveless tops and evening outfits with a jacket or over-blouse.

One-armed Biceps Curl

Strengthens and tones the front of your arm

Workout Prescription   Recommended weight 3–10 lb.
                                       10–15 reps, then switch sides. Do
                                       2–3 sets. Always remember to stretch
                                       before, during and after the exercise.

STARTING POSITION

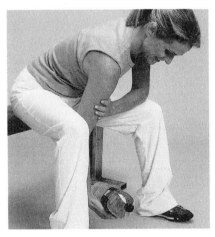

Working your Upper Body

Sit on the edge of a flat bench or a chair with your legs apart, your right elbow resting on your inner thigh. Rest your left forearm across the left thigh just above your knee and hold your right upper arm with your left hand. Holding a dumbbell (or half-litre bottle of water or tin of beans) in your right hand, palm up, let your right arm drop. With your shoulders square and abs contracted, lean forward slightly.

1   Keeping your body still, inhale and bend your right elbow, bringing the dumbbell up toward your chest, keeping your elbow on your thigh for stability.

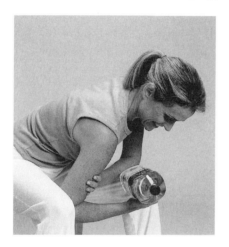

2   Exhale and return to the starting position. Repeat 10–15 times for each set.
3   Switch sides to work the left arm.

Tip

To make your workout that much harder, get three different weights: 10 lb, 5 lb and 3 lb dumbbells (or a litre bottle of water, 2 lb bag of sugar or can of beans). Start with the heaviest weight and curl until you achieve muscular failure (this means you are unable to do another rep). Immediately start another set with the next lightest pair. Go on until you cannot perform another rep. Pick up the lightest weight and, once again, go to muscular failure. Switch arms and repeat.

Fight Fat, Fight Fatigue

Single-arm Dumbbell Row

Tones and strengthens the upper back and front of the arms

Workout Prescription
1 set of 10–15 reps, working up to 3 sets of 10–20 reps.

STARTING POSITION

Bend at the waist so your back is parallel to the floor. Grasp a dumbbell with your right hand and place the left hand and knee on a bench or chair for back support. Your right foot forms a third point of a triangular stable base. This leg should be slightly bent and comfortable. Look forward and down.

1 Keeping your waist straight and leading with your elbow, pull the dumbbell to your chest, keeping your arm close to your body at all times.

83

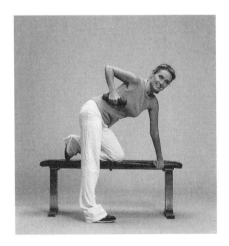

2 Pause briefly and lower, under control, until your arm is straight. Repeat for the desired number of reps.

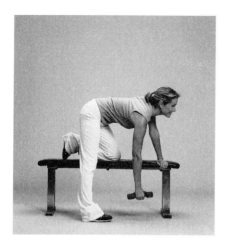

3   Change arms and repeat.

Tip

Avoid twisting your back during this exercise, and make sure it is supported at all times. Always lift and lower the dumbbell, tin of beans or bottle of water in a controlled manner.

TRICEPS – THE BACK OF YOUR ARM

Toning and strengthening your triceps muscle can minimize that annoying little jiggle on the back of your upper arm. What's more, strong triceps will better prepare you for everyday lifting tasks as well as sports moves such as a tennis backhand and swinging golf club. Many people tend to use complicated exercises when working their triceps. If they are using weights, they'll bring the weight up and twist it at the end of the movement, or they'll use weird rope exercises. It's just not necessary. The basic exercises I use have given me a great deal of success over the years with my clients – and can for you, too.

Triceps Dips

Tones and strengthens the back of the arm

Workout Prescription

1 set of 8–10 reps, working up to 3 sets of 10–20 reps. Make sure that the triceps tendon is fully warmed-up before starting.

STARTING POSITION

Sit on the edge of a bench with your legs extended forward, knees slightly bent, heels on the floor and toes up. Place your hands next to your buttocks, arms straight and palms down.

1   Keeping your torso erect and your hips under your shoulders, slide your buttocks off the bench until you're supporting your body weight with your arms (but don't lock your elbows).

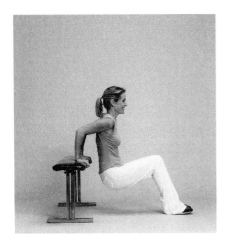

2   Now bend your elbows and lower your buttocks straight down towards the floor. Keep your back straight, hips close to the bench and chest open.

3   Straighten your arms to push yourself back up.

4   Repeat.

Tip

Keep your hips close to the bench. If you allow them to drift forward, you'll start to pull your shoulders forward as well. Don't sag into your shoulders.

Triceps Pull

Tones and strengthens backs of the arms (triceps) and shoulders

Workout Prescription   3 sets of 15–20 reps.

This exercise is a terrific triceps developer. Proper technique is the key here. It's important that the triceps tendon is fully warmed-up before starting. Always keep your back and shoulders rigid and tight, and make sure the triceps do the work.

This is a good exercise to do with a partner – one person supervises and then you switch roles.

1   Stand with your feet shoulder-width apart and hold a towel behind your back.

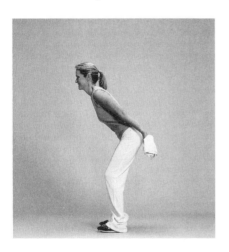

2   Lean forward from your hips with your knees slightly bent and your tummy tucked in.

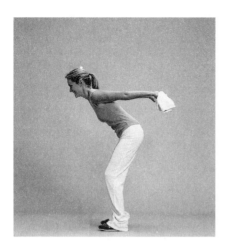

3 Keeping your arms straight, pull outwards on the towel and lift your arms
   behind you as high as you can. Try not to lean forward from the shoulders
   or waist. Hold the position for 5 seconds and lower again. Repeat.

Tip

Sometimes try and do the Triceps Pull with elbows in, other times with
elbows out. Changing elbow position allows you to feel the triceps working in a different way.

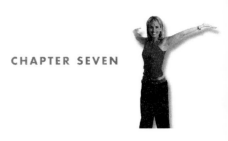

CHAPTER SEVEN

WORKING YOUR LOWER BODY

YOUR LOWER BODY

Your lower body includes your hips and bottom, your thighs – tops of thighs, back of thighs, inner and outer thigh – and your knee area.

For most women, the lower body is the most difficult area to keep fat-free and firm. It's often the first place that excess weight will sit – and stay – so these exercises are designed to help you shift weight and tone up in just the right places!

There are three main areas of the leg which present the toughest challenges:

1   Creating a distinct separation between the buttocks and the back of the leg.
2   Shaping the front thigh, specifically the area just above the knee.
3   Toning the inner thigh.

The following lower-body exercises address all these problem areas and provide many extra benefits: not only do well-conditioned legs look sleek and sexy, but the extra effort you put into your leg training translates into extra calories burned and a decrease in overall body fat.

Therefore, the more time spent working your lower body, the faster your weight loss, the leaner your physique and the greater your satisfaction from exercising.

The exercises that follow are carefully chosen to work, tone and strengthen precisely the right individual muscle groups to produce the shape you want. You should select 1–3 exercises from this chapter and perform them 3 times per week.

Remember:

1 *Don't work the same muscle groups two days in a row – without adequate recovery time you won't get the benefits and you might simply end up injured. So – pace yourself!*
2 *Always be sure to warm up before you start and to stretch and cool down each time you work out.*

Super Squat

Tightens, firms and adds shape to the front and inner thighs and buttocks, giving your legs a sleeker, firmer appearance

Workout Prescription   12–15 reps. Repeat 3 times.

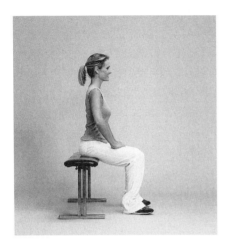

Sit on a chair or bench with your feet hip-width apart and point your toes straight ahead or angled slightly outwards, whichever feels more natural. Place your hands on your thighs, fingers facing each other.

91

1   On the count of 3, inhale and slowly raise yourself up from the chair, contracting your abs so your tailbone points down to the floor (when you stand up, your legs should be straight but relaxed).

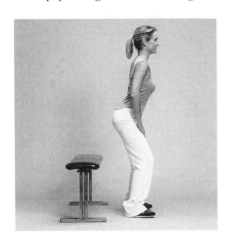

Working your Lower Body

2　On the count of three again, exhale and slowly lower yourself onto the chair or bench. Try keeping your weight back towards your heels, bending your hips and knees, and lowering your torso towards the floor. Your knees should always travel in the direction your toes are pointed and your hands must be kept on your thighs throughout this exercise.

3　Repeat.

Tip

If you find this way of squatting too easy, just let your buttocks touch the chair/bench but don't actually sit down.

Front Thigh Firmer

Tones and strengthens the top of your thighs and those flabby knees

Many people find it difficult to get rid of the flab around their knees. And the older you are, the harder it gets. It's ageing and makes the knee area look unattractive. For most of us, the only things standing between the body we want and the one we see in the mirror each morning are time and convenience. But you don't have to spend hours in the gym to get rid of droopy knees. Just a few minutes 3 times a week will do the trick.

Workout Prescription

15–20 repetitions on each side, building up to 3 sets of 20 reps.

STARTING POSITION

Sit on the floor with your back straight and your hands behind your buttocks for support (your fingers should be facing backwards). Extend your legs in front of you with your ankles flexed. Tuck your stomach muscles in tight.

1 Keeping your back straight, exhale and raise your left leg off the floor as high as possible without bending your knee.

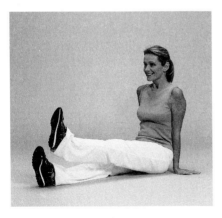

Working your Lower Body

2   Inhale and return to the starting position.

3   Repeat with the right leg.

Tip

With your toes raised and foot flexed, hold the end position for a count of 2 to increase the tension in your thigh. To increase the resistance and intensity even more, try adding ankle weights.

BACK OF THE THIGH – HAMSTRINGS

With bottoms being the new bosom and so many trendy tight-fitting trousers and skirts around, everyone wants to achieve that toned, sexy look. But few people realize how important it is to exercise the hamstrings as well as the buttocks. So far, it has been very hard to find a good hamstring toner – well, here it is!

Stiff-leg Deadlifts

Tones and strengthens the backs of your thighs and your buttocks

Workout Prescription

1 set of 10–15 reps, building up to 3 sets of 15–20 reps. Requires dumbbells or half-litre bottles of water or tins of beans.

95

STARTING POSITION

With your feet slightly apart, hold the dumbbells (or bottles of water/tins of beans) in front of your thighs.

1   Bend down and, keeping your legs straight and the dumbbells close to your legs, lower the dumbbells towards your shins. When they are in the lowest position, your butt should be pushed out behind your body as far as possible. This helps keep your back very flat, which is essential to the movement.

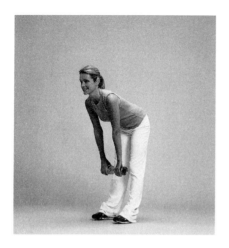

2 Stop when you feel a tightening at the back of your thighs and in your buttocks, then slowly return to the starting position and repeat. It is really important to stretch your legs for a long time after this workout.

Tip

The trick is to tuck your butt in and squeeze as you ascend from the bent-over position. If you keep the muscles in your lower back and along your spine very taut, you'll end up using the backs of your thighs and buttock muscles as the sole means of rising upwards.

Lunges

For buttocks, thighs and hamstrings

This is an exercise that works where you need help most. Just 3-minute sessions 2 or 3 times a week will give you curves where you used to have unsightly fat. It's a fact that extra weight stored on the hips, buttocks and thighs can be hard to budge – but it will go if you are willing to literally work your butt off!

Workout Prescription

1 set of 8–10 reps, building to 3 sets of 15–20. Alternate legs with each lunge.

STARTING POSITION
With your feet together, holding dumbbells in each hand, let your arms hang by your sides, palms in.

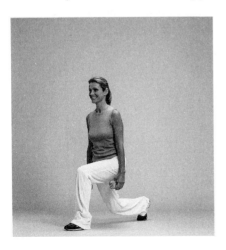

1   Inhale.
2   Exhale as you step forward with your left leg, leading with your heel.
3   Plant your foot down, bending your front knee directly over your ankle.

Working your Lower Body

4   Return to original position by pressing against your front heel and stepping back, never allowing your chest to fall forward.

Tip

Don't place stress on the knee by taking too short a step forward, forcing the knee to bend beyond your toes. Also, keep your abs tight and chest lifted throughout and your shoulders above your hips on the downward movement.

THE INNER THIGH

Are you embarrassed by your flabby, orange-peel, cellulite-coated inner thighs? Do you cringe when you need to wear trousers or shorts? Do your thighs rub together, creating a sore patch when you walk? If so, it's time to take some action.

Your Ultimate Leg Lift Series

A good all-rounder, progressively stimulating your butt and thighs to work even harder

To get that ultimate, sexy, Jennifer Lopez-style sculpted leg and shapely bottom that every woman craves, I have devised a series of leg lifts that vary in intensity. You'll see I've included a good, better and best version. They'll all make you stronger, since they all target the same muscles, but the better and best moves push you harder. Do the good version if you're tired or haven't been working out regularly and, when you're ready, try the next move. If you can't do it with good form, do as many reps as you can correctly, then drop to the previous level for the remaining sets. Switching things around is a terrific way to keep seeing results.

99

| Workout Prescription | 3 sets of 8–12 reps – and feel free to mix and match the moves. |

Good: Lying Leg Lift

STARTING POSITION

Lie on your left side. Bend your left arm and rest your head on your upper arm. Place your right hand in front of your chest, palm flat on floor. Bend your left knee to 90° and extend your right leg away from your front hip, turning your foot in so that your heel is higher than your toes.

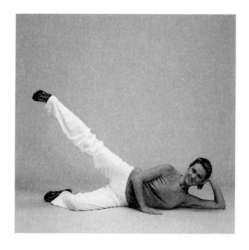

1   Squeeze your butt and raise your right leg slowly. Pull your abs in tight to stabilize your torso as your leg moves.
2   Switch sides and repeat with the left leg.

Why It's Good

You can isolate your butt with this leg movement; by rotating the thigh you target the less-often-used outer thigh muscle.

Better: Core Thigh Lift

STARTING POSITION

Begin on hands and knees, hands under your shoulders, back flat, knees
under your hips. Keep your neck in line with your spine and face down.
Place your left hand by your ear and open your elbow out to the side,
arm held at shoulder level.

1   Hold your abs tight to avoid tilting your hips as you squeeze your butt and
    lift your right knee to the side until your thigh is almost parallel to the
    floor. Maintain a 90° angle between thigh and calf.

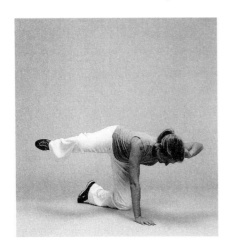

2   Slowly lower your leg back to floor, then repeat.
3   Finish all reps before switching sides and repeating.

Why It's Better

The face-down position adds the challenge of extra gravitational pull
while you balance. This makes your butt, back and abs work harder to
stabilize your body throughout the movement.

Best: Multidirectional Leg Raise

STARTING POSITION

Stand with your hands on your hips. Hold your abs tight to stabilize your pelvis.

1   Lift your rib cage high away from your hips as you lift your right leg and cross it in front of your left, leading with the instep, thigh turned outward, foot flexed.

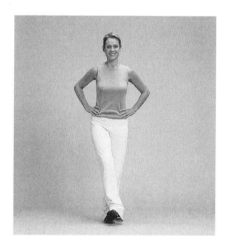

2   Squeeze your inner thighs to hold the leg in front of your body.

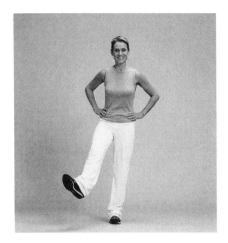

3 Squeeze your butt and move your right leg out away from your body, leading with the outside of your foot. Keep your hips stable and torso erect
   throughout.

4 Repeat, then switch sides.

Why It's Best

Standing legwork brings more muscle into the move. Not only is the
moving leg working, but your glutes work to stabilize your supporting
leg too. This exercise targets the inner and outer thighs as well as your
butt and abs.

Hot Legs

For the entire lower body: Tones and strengthens your midsection, butt, fronts and backs of your thighs and calves

This explosive move, which involves doing the Chubby Checker twist with a football between your legs, tones your midsection and strengthens every muscle in your lower body. It also gives you more power and agility for activities that require abrupt changes in direction, like skiing, tennis and soccer.

Workout Prescription

Warm up with 1 set of 8–10 reps at moderate effort. Rest for 30–40 seconds between sets. Then do a set of 8–10 reps at maximum effort. Build up to 5 all-out sets.

104

STARTING POSITION

Place a football between your knees. Stand with your knees bent 20°. Look straight ahead. Keep your elbows bent just below shoulder height.

1   Keeping your shoulders and head facing forward, jump and twist your lower body to the right, landing with your feet 30–90° off-centre.

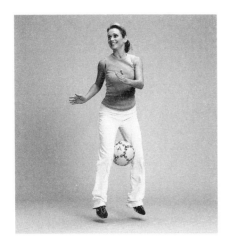

2   Immediately jump up and twist left, landing on the balls of your feet. Hop right and left, like a skier tackling moguls or pivoting round a tight turn. Squeeze the ball tightly with your inner thigh muscles.

3   Warm up with 1 or 2 sets of 8–10 reps at moderate effort. (Twisting right then left is 1 rep.) Rest a minute between sets. Then do a set of 8–10 reps at maximum effort, jumping as high and as quickly as you can. Build up to 5 all-out sets.

4   Do this exercise every fourth day – and expect soreness in your thighs, calves and butt at first.

Tip

Your goal is to twist fast. Imagine you're jumping on a hot plate and don't want your feet to stay on the floor long. Start with moderate effort and avoid looking down and rounding your spine, which can cause harm to your back. Instead, look straight ahead.

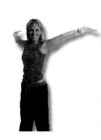

CHAPTER EIGHT

HOW TO ACHIEVE
the perfect butt!

G luteus medius – the 'Glutes'

A firm, tight bottom not only turns heads, but is a sure
sign of a well-conditioned body. The strong muscles of
the buttocks are our power centre, enabling us to
spring, jump and perform other dynamic moves.
Conditioned buttocks also help prevent knee and back
injuries. You can, to some extent, change the shape of
the posterior you were born with – and believe me,
there are as many types of butt as there are slang terms
for describing it. But no matter what that cheeky culprit,
heredity, has landed you with, diet and exercise can
help you make the very best of what you've got.

1. THE FLAT BUTT

If your butt is completely flat, it's never going to be a perfect peach. But since muscles determine shape, it's easy to add curves. Doing Squats *(see page 90)* with weights is a sure way to boost muscle. Or try this variation of a pelvic tilt:

Pelvic Tilt

Workout Prescription   1 set of 15 repetitions.

STARTING POSITION
Sit on the floor with knees bent, feet flat. Place your back against a low step and put your hands on the step, arms against the sides of your body, elbows back.

1   Contract your butt muscles to lift your pelvis 12 inches (30 cm).

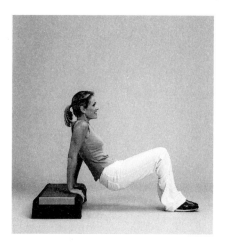

2   Hold for 10 seconds, then lower until your butt is 6 inches (15 cm) from floor.
3   Repeat 15 times.

2. THE BUBBLE BUTT

If your backside is of the shapely high variety (lucky you), the key is toning with low resistance.

Workout Prescription

To firm without bulk, avoid heavily-weighted squats. Instead, do lots of weight-free lunges *(see page 97)*. For a butt-slimming cardio workout, try walking, running or the elliptical trainer at your local gym.

3. THE PEAR-SHAPED BUTT

A narrow waist combined with 'saddlebags' makes for the curvaceous butt variety. Many women have this shape and most would love to put a stop to the droop. You can work wonders on a pear-shaped butt by combining regular fat-burning exercises like running or taking part in a 'Spinning' class at a gym, with leg presses *(see page 99)*. Also try this saddlebags toning move:

109

How to Achieve the Perfect Butt!

Saddlebags Toning

Workout Prescription   1 set of 15 repetitions. Switch legs
                                             and repeat.

STARTING POSITION

On hands and knees, flex your foot and push one heel straight back as if
to kick someone behind you.

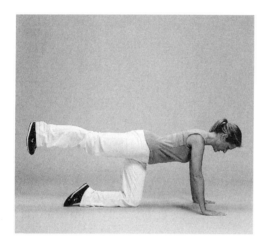

1   Keeping your leg straight, rotate from the hip, then flex your foot and point your toes forward as you slowly move your leg out to the side.

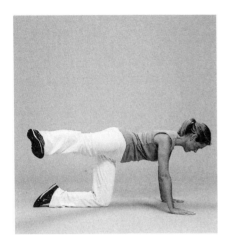

2   Lift up, then return to the starting position and repeat 15 times.
3   Switch legs.

4. THE RELAXED REAR

Skimping on glute work may cause you to lose muscle, making your butt hang low. Take this test: If you can hold a pencil in the butt-meets-leg crease, it's time to tighten up with some reverse lunges.

Reverse Lunge

Workout Prescription   1 set of 10 repetitions. Switch legs and repeat.

STARTING POSITION
Stand with your feet parallel, hip-width apart.

1   Step back with your left foot as far as you can, keeping the heel off the floor, and lower your body until your right knee bends 90°. Your back knee should bend but not touch the floor.

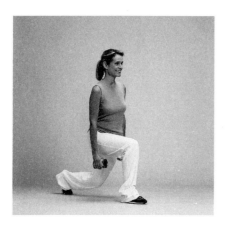

2   Squeeze your right buttock to stand, bringing your left leg to the starting position.
3   Repeat 10 times for each leg.

5. THE HEART-SHAPED BUTT

A lot of women have rears like an upside-down heart (quite similar to the pear-shaped, but more so). Pair this exercise with speed-walking, step classes or perhaps kickboxing to tone your hips and lift your butt.

Workout Prescription 1 set of 20 repetitions. Switch legs and repeat.

STARTING POSITION

Lie on your left side, knees bent so your thighs are perpendicular to your body.

1 Twist your upper body towards the floor so your forearms are flat in front of your chest on the floor.
2 Move your right knee just behind your left heel.
3 Keeping the knee bent, lift the top (left) leg 6 inches (15 cm), then lower.

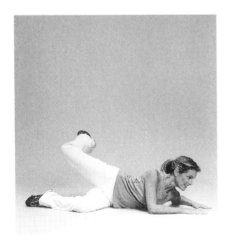

4 Repeat 20 times, then switch legs.

Sofa Squat

Tones and strengthens your buttocks and thighs, helps posture

You can do this at home, in a friend's home, in a hotel room if you're away on holiday or business – anywhere you happen to be. The motion chisels your buttocks and thighs and even helps you to stand straighter.

Workout Prescription   2 sets of 10–15 reps on each leg.

STARTING POSITION

Stand about 2 ft (60 cm) away from the armrest of your sofa, feet hip-width apart, facing away from the sofa.

1   Bend your left leg and place your foot flat against the armrest.
2   Squat back, pushing your butt towards the sofa and bending your right knee no deeper than 90°; hold, then squeeze your butt to straighten your right leg, returning to the upright position.

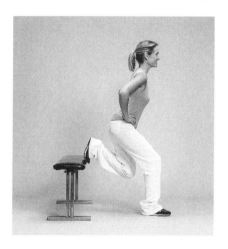

3   While standing, press your left foot back to the armrest, simultaneously squeezing your left butt muscle and thigh. Release and then lower to a half-squat again.

Tip

Don't place stress on your knee by taking too short a step forward, forcing your knee to bend beyond your toes. It's important to squat right back towards the sofa. Also, keep your abs tight and chest lifted throughout and your shoulders above your hips on the downward movement.

THE KICK BUTT WORKOUT

Strengthens and tones all the buttock muscles

   Do you need the kind of kick in the butt that only an instructor can give you? If so, these two simple bottom-blasting moves will whip yours into serious shape. All you need is a pair of light dumbbells (half-litre bottles of water or tins of beans will do).

Workout Prescription	1 set of 8–10 reps, building up to 3 sets of 12–15 reps, resting for 30–40 seconds between sets.

Back Kick

STARTING POSITION

Stand on your right leg with your left knee lifted in front of your body. Hold the dumbbells at waist height, palms facing your body. Bend your right knee into a semi-squat position. Make sure your right knee does not extend past your toes.

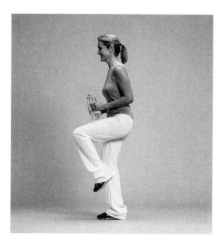

1 Now straighten your right leg as you extend your left leg straight behind you, left foot 3–6 inches (7.5–15 cm) off the floor. Hold the dumbbells close to your body throughout the move. Keep abs tight and try not to arch your back.

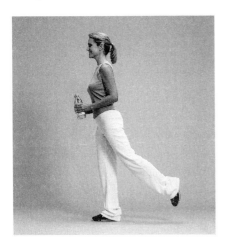

2 After one set, switch legs.

Tip
Clench your buttocks as you stand and kick back.

How to Achieve the Perfect Butt!

Side Kick

STARTING POSITION

Stand on your right leg, holding light dumbbells with your hands in front of you. Bend your right knee into a semi-squat position, keeping your left leg bent in front of your body. Make sure your right knee does not extend past your toes.

1 Now straighten your right leg while you raise your left leg to the side 45° from the floor, then slowly lower your left leg and squat on your right to return to the starting position.

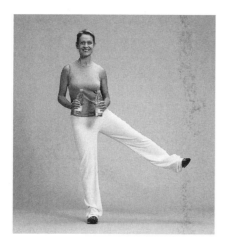

2 After one set, switch legs.

Tip
Hold your butt tight as you kick to the side.

The Perfect Plié

Tones and shapes the buttocks and backs of the thighs. Also tones the fronts of the thigh and, importantly, the inner thighs.

Borrow a move from ballet for the perfect all-round exercise for a shapely lower body. This is especially good for the inner thigh – a neglected area. The plié is a variation on the common strength-training squat. This turned-out stance targets the inner thighs and has been incorporated into countless exercise video routines, aerobics classes and strengthening programmes. It is a ballet move, however most non-dancers fail to follow the technique precisely, which can end up being dangerous for the knees. So, to do a safe, effective turnout, follow my directions carefully.

Workout Prescription	2 x 5 lb dumbbells required. When you can do 1 set of 12 reps with good technique, increase the weight.

119

STARTING POSITION

Stand with your feet slightly wider than shoulder-width apart, knees straight (not locked), abs in and tailbone pointing towards the floor. Hold the dumbbells with palms facing your thighs.

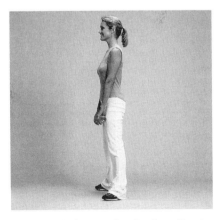

How to Achieve the Perfect Butt!

1. Shift your weight to your heels and rotate your feet and legs out from your hips as a unit, so that your knees and feet point towards the sides. Never let your feet turn out past your knees.

2. Shift your weight forward so that it's distributed evenly over the length of your feet. Slowly bend your knees and lower your body as far as you can, keeping your weight evenly distributed and your heels on the floor. Do not lower further than the point at which your thighs are parallel to the floor; don't let your knees extend past your toes or fall inward.

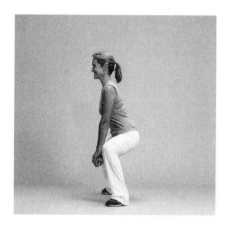

3. Slowly straighten your knees and raise your body to come back to the starting position.

4. As your strength increases, gradually increase the depth of your plié until your thighs are parallel to the floor. When you can do 12 pliés with good technique, increase the weight.

Tip

Throughout the move, keep your abdominal muscles tight and upper back lifted. Let your lower back maintain its natural curve, but avoid letting it arch further. Focus on the tailbone moving straight down and then straight up as your body is lowered and raised. If you feel knee discomfort, check your technique and try doing the exercise without holding any weights at all. Lower only as far as is comfortable.

Fight Fat, Fight Fatigue

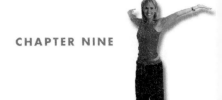

CHAPTER NINE

ALL NEW ABS

The core of your body includes your waist and midriff, your abdomen ('abs') and your internal pelvic muscles. Before you start work, remember: having a six-pack is more the result of a low body-fat percentage in the ab region than anything else. You could perform the perfect ab routine for a year, but if your diet isn't balanced and consistent, you will end up with a nice six-pack hiding under 2 inches of fat. This will only make your waist look thicker. So ab training without good nutrition only results in a strong but fat stomach.

121

Your abs are one of the easiest muscle groups to train anytime in your own home. Besides being aesthetically pleasing, a toned midsection is the core foundation of a healthy back, because strong abdominals will help give your torso the stability and support necessary to protect your back from injury.

First and foremost when doing this home-exercise programme, you want to make sure that you target the muscle group specifically by using correct form. Here are a few key points to remember:

SIX TOP TIPS FOR SUPER FIRM ABS

1. **Isolate your abdominal muscles** by relaxing your hip flexors (the muscle group in front of your hipbone) and concentrating on your abs doing all the work to curl your head and shoulder blades off the floor in upper-ab movements. Never anchor your feet underneath an object, as this will promote hip-flexor activity.

2. **Ensure proper form and spine alignment** by making sure your knees are bent and your feet are flat on the floor (or up). This helps protect your lower back. Place your hands lightly behind your head and look up towards the ceiling. To prevent neck pain, make sure your chin is far enough off your chest (you should be able to place your fist under your jaw).

3. **Make sure your lower back always remains in contact with the floor in upper-ab movements.** Crunch any higher than this and you'll use your hip flexor muscles to pull yourself up.

4. **Visualize your abdominal muscles** and concentrate on squeezing and holding the contraction at the top of the movement, focusing all your attention on the targeted region.

5. **Stretch your abs between sets to avoid cramping.** To do this, lie on your stomach (press-up position, palms on the floor, elbows next to your body) and press your pelvis into the floor while pushing through the palms of your hands to extend your arms (often called a *cobra stretch*). Make sure your pelvis remains in contact with the floor while you stretch your abs. Breathe deeply and relax your muscles further to increase the stretch.

6. **Practise proper breathing.** Exhale on the concentric phase of the crunch (rising up) and inhale on the eccentric portion of the crunch (lowering back down). Failure to breathe properly could cause cramping and dizziness and, in extreme cases, loss of consciousness.

Fight Fat, Fight Fatigue

ABS EXPRESS

Try these essential exercises for a marvellous midsection

This Abs Express programme takes only a few minutes and, if followed on a consistent basis along with a healthy diet, can help you develop the often-coveted set of washboard abs. You'll want to perform each of the following recommended exercises 3–4 days a week, aiming for 1–3 sets of 10–15 repetitions with 30 to 40-second rests between sets to begin with. As you become more advanced, increase the reps to the 20–25 range – but keep those rest periods the same. If you're doing it correctly you should find that 25–30 repetitions is the most possible in one set. If you can do more, you may need to tighten your form or increase your intensity by contracting hard at the top of each rep.

Remember:

1   *Don't work the same muscle groups two days in a row – without adequate recovery time you won't get the benefits and you might simply end up injured. So – pace yourself!*
2   *Always be sure to warm up before you start and to stretch and cool down each time you work out.*

Classic Crunch

Upper abs

1   Lie on your back with your knees bent and your feet flat on the floor, slightly apart.
2   With your hands opened behind your head, lift your upper body so that your shoulder blades clear the floor.

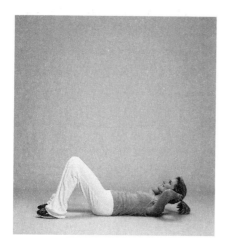

3   Breathe out as you lift and in as you release. Repeat 20 per set.

Frog Crunches

This exercise forces you to keep your lower abs contracted so your back doesn't arch

Workout Prescription

Start with 12–14 reps, building to 3 sets of 20.

1   Lie down on your back. Bend your knees and let them fall to the sides. Keep your feet together.
2   Next, hold your head with your hands and lift your chin away from your chest. Contract your stomach and slowly lift both shoulders off the floor.

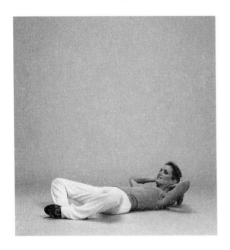

3   Rock your hips forward, pause at the top and lower back to the starting position.

Tip
To get the best isolation, always keep your lower back pressed into the floor. Try to move really slowly so you use more muscle fibres.

Lying Toe Touches

One of my favourites to make your upper abs really burn

Workout Prescription

Toe touches are challenging, so you might only be able to do 1 set of 10–15 reps.

1   Lie on your back and press the small of your back into the floor.
2   Extend your legs into the air and criss-cross your ankles in a scissors movement.
3   With your arms, reach towards your toes using your upper abs.

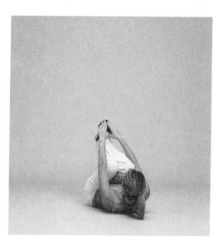

4   Pause at the top, then slowly lower back to start.

Tip

Sometimes try and use one arm at a time to slow the exercise down and really concentrate on the muscles doing the moving. If you feel any discomfort or strain in your lower back you should bend your knees, but make sure your hips and lower back remain on the floor.

One-leg V-crunches

A great way to target both the upper and lower abs

Workout Prescription   1 set of 10–15 reps.

1   In a basic crunch position, bend one knee so the foot is flat on the floor. Straighten the other leg, holding it a few inches off the floor.
2   Use your upper abs to raise your torso. Squeeze your lower abs and bring your knee as close to your face as you can, while keeping your lower back pressed into the floor.

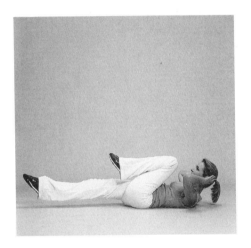

3   Flex your abs at the top and return to the start.
4   Switch legs and repeat.

Tip
Never let your shoulders or leg touch the floor. Try to keep your abs contracted throughout the entire exercise.

Five-step Crunch

Overall abs

1   In your classic crunch position, reach your arms forward with your palms facing the sky (up). Lift your body so that your hands reach over your knees, and hold.

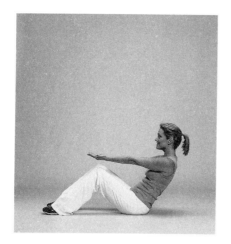

2   Extend your arms directly over your head and hold.

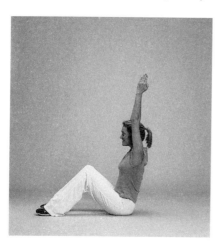

Fight Fat, Fight Fatigue

3 Reach three 'steps' upwards, lifting 1 inch higher every step, and then release back down to the floor.
4 Repeat 10–15 per set.

GOOD CRUNCH TECHNIQUE

Many people complain that crunches cause neck pain, but this will only occur if you make the mistake of yanking on your head. Another major crunching error: lifting your torso straight off the floor, as opposed to curling it upward. How do you know whether you're curling or just lifting? When you do a crunch, freeze at the top of the movement. You should not be able to draw a straight line through the part of your back that's lifted off the floor; instead, your torso should be in a slightly rounded, almost C-shaped position. As you advance, slow the movement or hold a light weight with both hands on top of your head.

THE HIGH VARIETY ABS PLAN

Here is a series of stomach and midriff exercises that, when combined, offer an interesting spin on classic ab exercises which, more than likely, you haven't ever considered before. Implementing pauses will definitely retrain your ab muscles. So, if you've been using steady reps as your technique, mix it up. Another twist to this routine is the addition of a ball, which will inspire you and also add an element of thought to your workout. Try this routine for at least three weeks – I dare you not to notice a difference!

Workout Prescription

Do 1 set of each exercise from the Variety Plan, or choose to focus on 3, performing 3 sets of each. Always rest for 30–40 seconds between sets and always include the stretch as part of your workout.

1. Ab Stretch

Start and finish with this stretch

1 Lie face down with your hands directly under your shoulders. Keep your legs extended (turning your feet outward will enhance the stretch).

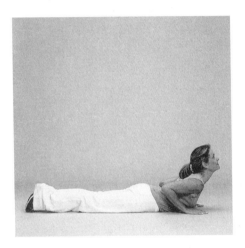

131

2 Slowly raise your upper body by pressing with your hands, extending your arms and raising your head and shoulders upward. Look up to the sky and hold for about 15 seconds. Let the abs stretch and then release.

2. Reverse Crunch

Lower abs

1 Lie on the floor with your feet in the air, knees bent about 45°.
2 Keeping your hands by your sides and your shoulders on the floor, pull your knees in so that your hips lift slightly off the floor. Move slowly through the range of motion.

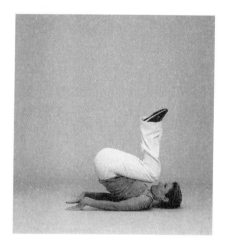

3 Repeat 12 times per set.

3. Ball Balanced Crunch

Overall abs

1 Position yourself as if you were going to perform a classic crunch, but instead of resting your feet on the floor or on a chair, place your feet on a ball.

2 With your hands behind your head, with opened fingers, exhale as you slowly lift your head and shoulders off the floor, keeping your feet on the ball.

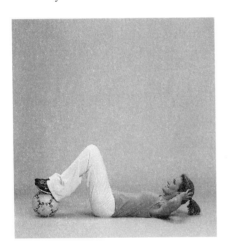

3 Release and repeat for 15 reps per set.

4. Ball Press

Upper abs

1 Holding on to a ball, hold your body in a classic crunch position.
2 Press the ball upward towards the ceiling. As your arms extend, lift your upper body until your shoulders are off the floor.

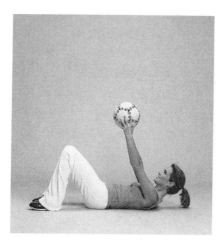

3 Repeat 12 times per set.

5. Basic Weighted Sit-up

Tones and strengthens all your stomach muscles

The key to creating a strong, defined midsection is full range of motion for the spine. This exercise is perfect, as it works several muscle groups together to create a compound movement. As a result, this one exercise will tone and strengthen the top, bottom and sides of your stomach.

When you perform the full sit-up, only do this with a rolled-up towel under your lower back. Make sure you concentrate on the ab movement and don't pull or strain your neck or head. Use your abs to pull your torso over the mat or towel and then continue into a full sit-up. When you reverse direction, simply uncurl your torso in a controlled manner to return to the starting position. Nothing could be easier. And note, this routine shows you how to change from a Michelin man to a bikini babe by using time, rather than reps, to keep it intense.

135

Workout Prescription

Perform this exercise for 5–15 seconds until you feel a burn in your abs, then rest and repeat 3 more times. As you become stronger, increase the time of each set.

STARTING POSITION

Lie flat on your back with your knees bent at about 45°. Do not anchor your feet, but keep your heels on the floor. Place a mat under your lower back for firm support as your spine curls during the sit-up movement. Holding a dumbbell in both hands (half-litre bottles of water will do), place your hands between your legs.

1 Begin the sit-up motion, curling the spine forward by contracting your abdominal muscles, pulling you over the mat into a straight plane. As you continue the curling movement, your pivot point changes to the hip area. This is where your ab muscles reach the end of their strength curve and your lower internal waist muscles help to complete the final contraction of your abs to your pelvis.

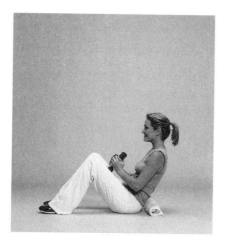

2 When you lie back down, just uncurl, reversing the sit-up movement.

Tip

Do not jerk your body up or use momentum to increase your range of motion or repetition total. Concentrate on tight contraction of your ab muscles and go on until you cannot do another rep.

Remember to repeat the Ab Stretch (*page 131*) as the final part of this workout.

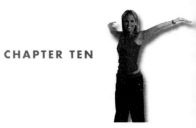

CHAPTER TEN

TARGET YOUR BODY TYPE

N ow that you know how to workout, you can select a plan designed specifically for your body type. Thin but flabby? Fat but fit? Not all workouts are equally effective for all body types. This chapter explains what will be most effective for *you* – isolating the key moves and routines that will best meet your needs and help you to achieve your goals.

We're talking about the varying body shapes, levels and ratios of body fat and muscle tone that make real women differ. Here, we've identified the three key real-life body types – Kiwis, Pears and Apples – and provided the perfect exercise and food prescription for each one.

Each plan starts with tailored-to-you versions of the core strength moves, plus two unique moves for your body type. In addition to the basic core strength work, your body type exercise prescription contains windows which you'll fill with workouts of your own choice, based on the cardio recommendations necessary for your type to achieve your fitness goals safely. You can use heart rate or, more simply, our Exertion Scare to check how hard you're working!

Remember always to warm up, stretch and cool down.

HOW HARD ARE YOU WORKING?

Customize your cardio sessions by exercising at the right intensity.

Light	You're moving slowly; you can speak with ease.
Moderate	You're slightly breathless but can still talk.
Somewhat Hard	You're breathing fast.
Very Hard	You're panting and exercising vigorously.

BASIC BODY STRENGTH EXERCISES

See your body type prescription later in this chapter for extra detail about how much and how often you should perform these exercises for your individual body type routine.

Some of these exercises require weights. As always, if you haven't got dumbbells, you can always use half-litre bottles of water or tins of beans.

MOVE	HOW TO DO IT
Squats	Stand with your feet shoulder-width apart; bend your knees to 90°, weight on your heels. Squeeze your butt to stand; repeat.
Lunges	Stand with your feet hip-width apart. Take a wide step back; land softly. Lower your hips until the front knee is at 90°. Squeeze your butt to stand. Switch legs.

Fight Fat, Fight Fatigue

Step-ups	Step up onto a step with your right foot; bring your left leg up. Step down with your right foot, then left. Switch legs and repeat.
Push-ups	Start on your hands and knees, hands shoulder-width apart. Extend your legs straight behind you and balance on your hands and toes with your body in a straight line. Bend your elbows to lower your chest to the floor, then straighten to push up. Repeat.
Chest press	Lie on your back with your knees bent; hold weights by your chest, palms forward. Push up over your chest to straighten your arms. Lower and repeat.
Rows	Sit in a chair, feet flat on the floor. Lean forward with a straight back. Hold weights beside your ankles, palms in. Pull your elbows up and behind. Lower, then repeat.
Overhead press	Sit in a chair, feet flat. Hold weights by your shoulders, palms facing forward. Push your hands up to straighten your arms. Lower and repeat.
Biceps curls	Sit or stand. Hold weights by your sides, palms forward. Lift weights to your shoulders, elbows by your sides. Lower and repeat.

139

Target your Body Type

Ab twists	Lie on your back, knees bent, feet flat, hands behind your head. Raise your shoulders 3–6 inches (7.5–15 cm) off the floor, then rotate your rib cage to each side. Lower and repeat.

FOR KIWIS

YOUR BODY

There's no hiding the fact that you have weight to lose. You're well proportioned, but when it comes to exercise, you tire easily and feel uncoordinated.

YOUR WORKOUT

Take small steps that you can accomplish easily.

FOCUS ON

Building stamina with easy-to-master activities like walking and cycling, performed at low intensity – incorporating intervals (higher-intensity bursts) into cardio sessions to boost calorie burn – using light weights – developing torso stability.

Don't Do

Hard workouts – complicated fitness classes – sports that require advanced skills. You should begin simply, instead of burning yourself out too soon.

Kiwi Workout Plan

CORE EXERCISES

How much weight	1 lb to 5 lb dumbbells
How often	2 times a week
How hard	1 set, 10–15 reps

CARDIO

How long	Easy sessions: 35–45 minutes
	Interval sessions: 20 minutes
How often	Easy: 3 times per week. Intervals:
	1 time per week
How hard	Easy, light-intensity intervals, alternate
	30 seconds at moderate with 3
	minutes at light intensity

FOR BALANCE AND CONTROL

A   Stand with your feet hip-width apart and parallel, arms by your sides. Slide your left foot up your right calf to the knee. At same time, raise your arms; stop at shoulder level. Hold for 30 seconds; build to more if you can. Lower and repeat on other leg.

B   In the same standing position, hold weights in front of your thighs, palms facing your body. Raise your left leg at the back and your right arm in front to shoulder level. Hold for 15 seconds (build up to longer); lower. Switch sides.

FOR CARDIO AND MUSCLE POWER

A   Stand with your feet slightly wider than hip-width, toes pointing forward. Bend your knees and lower your hips to knee level. Support your hands on your thighs.

Target your Body Type

B   Gather energy by lowering your body slightly, then squeeze your butt and thighs to jump, opening your legs into a straddle and raising your arms to the sides. Land softly, shifting your body weight to your heels. Jump 4 times.

FOR PEARS

YOUR BODY

Your upper body looks great in clothes, but your butt is much lower than you'd like. Your thighs are far too wide, your posture could improve and some body parts jiggle more than they should.

YOUR WORKOUT

Pump up the intensity of what you do. For strength moves, try to over-load the muscles you target as much as possible while maintaining good alignment.

FOCUS ON

Building muscle with high-resistance cardio work such as cycling, power-walking, elliptical training, stair-climbing and swimming. You should also work on improving your posture.

Don't Do

Long, low-intensity cardio workouts. The muscles in your lower body have to be challenged to change. Staying at low intensity just won't do the trick!

Pear Workout Plan

CORE EXERCISES

How much weight   5 to 10 lb dumbbells
How often   3 times a week
How hard   2 sets, 8–12 reps

CARDIO

How long   30 to 45-minute sessions
How often   3–5 times per week
How hard   Moderate to somewhat hard

FOR LOWER BODY STRENGTH

A   Place your right foot on a step. Hold weights by your sides, arms straight.

B   Squeeze your butt and step up on your left foot; push your straight right leg back. Keep your abs tight and move with control. Lower your leg, then repeat on the other side.

FOR LOWER BODY SHAPING

A   Stand with your feet parallel, hip-width apart. Hold weights in front of your thighs, palms facing your body.

B   Step back as far as possible with your left foot (back heel off the ground) and raise both arms in front of you to shoulder level. Contract the butt of the front leg and return to standing. Repeat, alternating legs.

143

Target your Body Type

FOR APPLES

YOUR BODY

You don't have much stamina and strength and you carry extra body fat around your middle. You would like to lose that spare tyre, sculpt the rest of your body and get fit.

YOUR WORKOUT

Maximize the calorie burn by upping the fat-burning engine in your body with weight workouts and cardiovascular exercise.

FOCUS ON

Working at a higher intensity during cardio. Try running the elliptical trainer and multi-impact aerobics – harder strength moves and abdominal exercises.

Don't Do

The same old routines and low-intensity workouts. To make a real difference you need to get sweaty and introduce some more variety to your workouts.

Apple Workout Plan

CORE EXERCISES

How much weight	5 to 10 lb dumbbells
How often	3 times a week
How hard	2 sets, 10–15 reps

CARDIO

How long	Longer sessions: 40–60 minutes
	Interval sessions: 35–45 minutes

Fight Fat, Fight Fatigue

How often	Long: 2 or 3 times per week
	Intervals: 2 times per week
How hard	Long: Moderate intensity. Intervals:
	Alternate 2 minutes somewhat hard
	with 3 minutes moderate

FOR A LEANER UPPER AND LOWER BODY

A   Stand with your feet shoulder-width apart, toes forward. Hold weights by your thighs. Squat by lowering your hips, keeping your body weight on your heels. Bend your elbows to bring the weights to your shoulders, palms facing your body.

B   Exhale and squeeze your butt to stand up, pushing the weights overhead. Hold, then lower and repeat.

FOR TORSO STABILITY AND ABS

145

A   Lie on your back, knees bent, feet flat. Pull in your abs to stabilize your back, then lift your shoulders, reaching your arms overhead. Lift your right foot slowly, bringing your thigh to your chest. Hold, then lower the foot and switch legs.

B   With your arms and shoulders still lifted, raise your left knee to your chest. Keeping the left knee lifted, slowly pulse your right foot, then switch sides. Tighten your abs throughout the move. If your neck tires, bring your hands behind your head for support.

TAILOR-MADE FOR SHORTER AND TALLER WOMEN – WHY YOUR SIZE MATTERS

Finding moves that match your height could take your workout to new levels.

In the previous section I showed you how to prescribe exercises to suit your body type, but you should also consider your height, something that is rarely taken into account. If you're fairly short or tall, your body may be getting in the way. Being above or below average height can put you at a biomechanical disadvantage when you exercise. Some exercises require movements that compromise benefits or cause injury. Try the following substitutions.

If You're 5 ft 10 or Above

SKIP: SQUATS

Tall women absorb more pressure in the lower back, which can be dangerous while trying to keep their spine straight during squats.

Instead, try:

Dumbbell Lunge Pull

This move won't put pressure on the spine

Workout Prescription   1 set of 8–10 reps, building up to 3 sets of 16–20 reps.

STARTING POSITION
Stand with feet hip-width apart. Hold a light dumbbell (half-litre bottle of water or tin of beans) in each hand, by your sides, palms in.

1   Lunge back with your left leg. As you step back, extend both arms forward at hip level.

2   With your left leg still behind you, straighten both legs; simultaneously pull your elbows behind your ribs and squeeze your shoulder blades together.

3   Slowly lower and repeat, switching legs.

4   For an advanced option, in position (2) bring your left knee up to waist level.

Tip

When lunging, step back far enough to land on your toes, not your heels. Bend your front knee to a 90° angle, making sure you keep your knee directly above your ankle. Return to the starting position. Repeat with the left leg.

SKIP: HANGING KNEE AND LEG RAISES

Longer thighs extend further from the body when raised up than shorter thighs do, straining the hip flexors and lower back.

Instead, try:

Tuck Curls

Workout Prescription   1 set of 8–10 reps, building up to 3 sets of 15–20 reps.

STARTING POSITION

Lie down on your back with a towel rolled into a long sausage shape under the base of your skull. Keep hold of each end of the 'sausage'.

1   Bring your knees as close to your chest as you can, crossing your ankles (your legs should be completely relaxed). Pressing your abs in towards your back, take a deep breath and exhale.

2   As you lift, curl your spine up to bring your rib cage and pelvis towards each other. Keep the movement slow and controlled.

Target your Body Type

3   Return to the starting position and repeat.

Tip

Try to keep in mind while performing tuck curls that it's the tightening and flattening action of your abs that bring your rib cage and pelvis towards each other.

If You're a Woman 5 ft 2 or Under

SKIP: LEG CURL MACHINES

Shorter women's hips bend before the curve in the bench, forcing them to shift further back on the machine, which stresses the back.

Instead, try:

Straight-leg Dumbbell Deadlifts

148

Tones and strengthens the backs of your thighs and buttocks

(This exercise targets the hamstrings effectively, but it's easier on your lower back.)

Workout Prescription   1 set of 10–12 reps, building up to
3 sets of 15–20 reps.

STARTING POSITION

Stand tall with your feet shoulder-width apart, contracting your abdominals hard. With your arms hanging down, hold a 5 to 10 lb weight in front of your thighs, palms facing your body.

1   Contract your butt muscles, keeping your knees straight (not locked) and slowly bend forward at the waist. Lower your body comfortably until the weights are as near to the floor as you can get them.
2   Use your leg and butt muscles to rise again to a full standing position.

Tip

The trick is to tuck your butt in and squeeze as you ascend from the bent-over position. If you keep the muscles in your lower back and along your spine very taut, you'll end up using the backs of your thighs and buttock muscles as your sole means of rising upward.

SKIP: CHEST-PRESS MACHINES

The handles on these machines tend to be spaced too far apart for shorter women to grasp, which can cause elbow and shoulder strain.

Instead, try:

Dumbbell Press with Weights

Tones and strengthens backs of the arm, front shoulders and chest
(Without the locked-grip position, you can keep your hands directly in line with your elbows.)

(149)

Workout Prescription	1 set of 10–12 reps, building up to 3 sets of 15–20 reps.

STARTING POSITION

For your chest, lie on a bench or floor with your knees bent, feet flat on the bench or floor and a weight in each hand.

1 With your palms facing forward, push the weights upward until your arms are extended above your chest, keeping your elbows directly below your hands and even with your shoulders.
2 Lower the weights along the sides of your chest. Then push the weights back up again and repeat.

Tip

If you are using a proper gym bench, as a variation to the above:

A   For the upper chest, set the bench at a 45° incline and lie with your head at the highest point and your feet on the floor.

B   For the lower chest, set the bench lower and lie with your head at the lowest point of the bench and your feet flat on the floor.

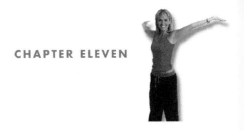

CHAPTER ELEVEN

QUICKIE WORKOUTS

Y ou can get slimmer and fitter – *fast*. As with anything worth having, the old saying 'No pain, no
gain' applies here. You do have to put in that extra
effort – but you will be repaid by achieving your goal.
Here are some quickies I've devised specially for all
areas of the body that will get you real results in just
two weeks – and my speedy tips on how to have you
looking and feeling great today!
Party tonight? Try this…

151

RESCUE REMEDY BODY TONE
AND CONFIDENCE BOOSTER

**An all-over body workout to look leaner and feel great in just a few
minutes**

If you happen to be carrying a few extra pounds and you'd love
to wear something more sexy and revealing, but you need a bit of a

confidence boost, read on. It's a well-kept secret that I tell my celebrity clients just before they go on stage: a few key exercises will give the body instant tone and definition. Not only will you look more defined, glowing and energized, but these moves will also calm your nerves, recharge your batteries and give you that crucial, last-minute confidence boost.

THE WORKOUT

You'll need a skipping rope.

The first move gets your heart rate pumping.

The strength move that follows allows your heart rate to dip slightly.

Then you pick up the pace again with a kickboxing move and perform the final anaerobic burst all-out.

When you've finished, march in place until your heart rate has slowed down.

Then stretch thoroughly.

152

Skipping Jog

| Beginners | 2–4 minutes |
| Intermediate/Advanced | 2–6 minutes |

Keep your feet shoulder-width apart, knees slightly bent, and grasp the rope handles in each hand. Start a basic two-foot jump, hopping on both feet at the same time with no in-between bounce. Then, with each rope turn, lift one foot off the floor as if you were jogging. Alternate. Land on the balls of your feet, but let your heels touch down.

Boxer's Press-up

| Beginners | 15–20 reps |
| Intermediate/Advanced | 25–30 reps |

Come to the press-up position *(see page 65)*, knees on floor, torso in a straight line. Extend your right arm out to the side, palm flat. Reach your left hand in front of your shoulder. Keep your toes on the floor, abs tight, and bend your elbow to lower your chest to the floor without arching your back. Hold, then straighten your arm to push up. Repeat for half the reps before switching arms.

Punch-kick Side

| Beginners | 1–3 minutes |
| Intermediate/Advanced | 2–6 minutes |

1 Stand with your left foot forward, knees soft. Bring your left arm out just under shoulder level, elbow bent so your fist is 6–12 inches (15–30 cm) from your face, palm in, elbow pointing to the floor. Keep your right fist by your ear in the resting phase. Punch with your left fist straight out to the side at shoulder height, forearm parallel to floor and wrists straight. Retract your left hand before you kick.

2 Immediately after you punch, bend your left knee and raise your thigh out to the side, turning your left hip slightly forward and flexing your left foot as you kick it out. (Keep your right knee bent.) Push out with your leg by leading with the heel, stopping when your left foot is about 12 inches (30 cm) off the floor. Avoid high kicks until your hamstrings are flexible enough to do them safely and you have learned to execute this movement with control. Kick with force, but avoid locking the knee.

3 Kick for 10–15 seconds, then switch sides and repeat. Continue to alternate sides for the rest of the exercise.

153

Anaerobic Burst — Foot Fire

| Beginners | 30–60 seconds |
| Intermediate/Advanced | 60–90 seconds |

Stand with your feet hip-width apart, toes pointing forward. Start jogging on the spot at a normal pace, then speed up to jog at double time. Your toes should make a rapid pitter-patter motion. Then move your legs alternately in an out-out, in-in pattern. Your arms can drum in front of you or just hang. Increase the intensity by moving your feet faster.

JUST 10 MINUTES!

Ultra quick all-over muscle toning and metabolic boost

Got 10 minutes? Well, here's a bite-sized fitness routine that will get you into that little black dress – fast!

You can perform this workout in your home or behind closed doors at your office. The exercises are quite intense and work several muscle groups simultaneously, so you get the greatest benefit in the shortest amount of time. (Although they are not meant to replace your regular total-body exercise regime, they will give you fast results, prevent backsliding and keep your metabolism humming all day long.)

For maximum benefit, do as many repetitions of the exercise as you can in the time allotted, using the proper form.

1 MINUTE: JUMPING JACKS OR JOGGING ON THE SPOT

This will warm you up and get your body going. Do as many as you can in the allotted time.

3 MINUTES: DESK PUSH-UPS

Stand 2–4 ft (60–120 cm) from a sturdy desk and lean forward, legs and feet together, placing your hands slightly more than shoulder-width apart on the desk. Bend your arms to lower yourself and hold. Straighten your arms to return to starting position.

3 MINUTES: SQUATS WITH CALF RAISES

Stand with your feet more than hip-width apart, keeping your hands on your hips, and bend your knees. Lower yourself as far as you can without letting your knees go past your toes. When you come up from the squat, lift both heels to stand on the balls of your toes. Lower your heels to the floor, then go back into the squat. Repeat.

2 MINUTES: PELVIC TILT CRUNCHES

Lie on your back with your hands loosely laced behind your neck and your knees bent. Tighten your abs and curl forward until your shoulders are about 2 inches off the floor. Don't touch your chin to your chest. As you come up, tilt your pelvis towards you to work the lower ab muscles and buttocks as well. Lower your pelvis and shoulders. Repeat.

1 MINUTE: BEND OVER AND STRETCH

This will help loosen your lower back, hamstrings and calves. Take a wide stance, feet more than hip-width apart, and grasp each elbow with the opposite hand. Bend over as far as you can go, keeping your knees slightly bent and taking deep breaths.

SUPER SEXY SHOULDERS WORKOUT

Strengthens and tones your deltoids (shoulders) in a flash

Like Catherine Zeta Jones, you can be happy, healthy, toned and look fabulous just weeks after giving birth. Her bosom and shoulders are particularly stunning – and you can get Catherine's erogenous shoulders if you follow this speedy plan to get yourself back in tone fast. It works equally well even if you've let yourself go a bit. So if you are short on time but would love sexy shoulders, then this is an exercise designed for you!

Stand with feet shoulder-width apart, knees slightly bent, chin pointed forward. Hold a pair of 3 to 5 lb dumbbells (tins of beans or half-litre bottles of water will do) in front of your pelvis, palms facing each other, elbows in line with shoulders.

1 Rotate your palms out to face forward as you raise the dumbbells out to your sides to shoulder level. Continue raising your arms until the dumbbells are above your head.

2 Lower arms, turning wrists so that your palms face each other at the starting position.

3 Repeat the move 3–5 times.

SEXY ARMS WORKOUT

Tones the deltoids, biceps and triceps

There's no doubt that a quick glimpse of Angela Bassett, Madonna, Sandra Bullock, Sheryl Crow or Sarah Jessica Parker confirms that arm muscles look good. These women's upper arms are practically living anatomy diagrams, with clearly defined deltoids (the muscle that caps the shoulder), biceps (along the front of the arm) and triceps (along the back of the arm). If you want arms like them, you can get them in 6 weeks – if you persevere. It's up to you.

Workout Prescription

Do these 3 upper-body exercises 3 times a week, resting a day between workouts. All levels can do the same number of sets and repetitions, but adjust the weight according to your fitness level.

Three-way Shoulder Raises

STARTING POSITION

Stand with feet hip-width apart, 5 to 10 lb dumbbells in each hand (half-litre bottles of water or tins of beans will do).

1 Bend your elbows slightly; lift your arms sideways to shoulder height.
2 Bend your knees; lean forward with your back close to parallel to the floor, arms down. Lift your arms out to shoulder height.
3 Do 3 sets of 10 reps in each position. Rest 45–60 seconds between sets.

Decline Press-ups

STARTING POSITION

Place your knees on a step, your hands on the floor, with your arms straight in line with your shoulders. Keep your body straight from head to tailbone.

157

1 Bend your elbows, lowering your torso until your elbows are about in line with your shoulders. Press up.
2 Do 3 sets of 10–15 reps. Rest for 45–60 seconds between sets.

Concentration Curls

STARTING POSITION

Sit with a 5 to 10 lb dumbbell (half-litre bottle of water or tin of beans will do) in your right hand, resting the back of your upper arm against your inner thigh. Lean forward with your back straight and abs contracted.

1 Bend your right elbow, bringing the dumbbell towards your right shoulder. Do reps. Switch hands.

Quickie Workouts

2   Do 3 sets of 12–15 reps per arm. Decrease the weight by 5 lb each set.

Tip

Always remember to warm up, cool down and stretch with 3–5 minutes of light cardio work, such as marching on the spot.

CLEAVAGE WORKOUT

Create great curves and give your bust a boost

If you feel – and look – a bit jaded and droopy, all you need are my six sensational 'cleavage-creating' exercises.

Warm up by jogging or marching lightly on the spot, with your feet never more than a foot or so off the floor. Continue for up to 2 minutes, then commence the exercises.

For the three where no weights are involved, the repetition range should be 3 sets of 20–25 reps.

For the other three exercises, use 3 to 5 lb weights or half-litre bottles of water or tins of beans. Do 3 sets of 8–12 reps, resting for 60 seconds between sets.

Don't forget: **Always stretch after exercising.**

Level: Easy

PECKS APPEAL

Standing or sitting, bring your arms up in front of you at chest level, elbows parallel to shoulders. Grasp your left forearm with your right hand and your right forearm with your left hand. Alternately, push and relax, squeezing your chest muscles together while gradually raising your elbows and hands towards your forehead. You should feel your chest muscles working and see your boobs rising. Pushing continuously, bring your arms down to abs level.

PECKS PUMP

Stand straight with your arms crossed in front of your chest and your hands fisted. Keeping your arms bent, slowly extend your elbows out behind you. Pause, then return to the starting position.

KNEEL AND CLAP

Kneel with your arms out in front, palms facing each other shoulder-width apart. Slowly clap your hands together. Return to the starting position, then pass your right arm over your left. Pause, then return to the starting position. Clap again, then pass the left arm over the right. This all equals one repetition.

Level: Intermediate

CHEST CROSS

Stand with your feet just wider than hip-width, toes pointing forward. Holding weights, cross your arms in front of your hips, palms facing down, elbows slightly bent. Lean forward 45°, back straight. Tighten your abs and your lower back muscles. Slowly arc your arms, pulling the weights out and up to the sides by bending and lifting both elbows. Stop when your elbows are in line with your shoulders, hands in front of your elbows, palms facing down. Contract your chest muscles as you retract your arms and retrace the path very slowly back to crossed position. Remember to keep your elbows slightly bent as you move your arms.

Level: Intermediate/Advanced

REVERSE PRESS

Lie on a bench or the end of a bed, your legs extended over your hips, knees slightly bent. Holding weights, open your arms out to the sides, elbows bent 90° at shoulder level, palms facing towards your feet. Push your arms up above your chest to straighten your elbows as you contract

159

your abs so that your pelvis tilts forward, moving your legs over your waist. Hold the position, then lower your arms and hips slowly.

Level: Advanced

ASSISTED PRESS-UP

Place a rolled-up mat or large towel on the floor. Get in a press-up position with the mat or towel just under your hips. Bend your elbows and lower your chest to floor. Hold your hips, shoulders and heels in line. Exhale and push up. Keep your abs tight throughout. As you get stronger, place the mat/towel under your thighs, then shins, then finally remove it. If your shoulders or wrists feel uncomfortable, then shift your body weight back onto your feet.

THE BLUE JEANS QUICKIE

Tone your butt and belly and slide back into those sexy blue jeans

You won't throw them away, even if you can't get into them any more. They're lurking at the back of your wardrobe to remind you of the sexy lean machine you used to be. And even if you can just about lever yourself into them after a marathon and soul-destroying seam-straining, zipper-complaining, red-faced struggle, you look like the side of an oil tanker. I'm talking about your favourite 501s. But gals, there's hope – follow this fat-busting quickie and it won't be your blue jeans that will bust, but your flab from the places where it counts the most. While it's true that you can't spot-reduce, lowering body fat overall means you'll shed it fastest where you store it – and in most women, that's the abs, hips and thighs.

Workout Prescription   All 3 sets of 8–12 reps per exercise
                                     at least twice a week.

Single Leg Squat

Targets the front and back of your thighs

STARTING POSITION
Balance on your right foot, leg straight but not locked. To help you balance, bend your left leg slightly and shift your left thigh back so that it is slightly behind your hip. Hold bent elbows by your sides, hands at waist level.

1 Push your hips back as you slowly bend your right knee and lower body until your knee is at about a 90° angle. Reach both arms straight in front of your hips. Hold, then squeeze your right buttock to straighten up.
2 Pull your elbows back as you stand, squeezing your shoulder blades together.
3 Repeat, then switch sides.

161

Single Leg Deadlift

Targets butt and back of the thighs

STARTING POSITION
Stand on your left leg and press your right toe to the floor. Rest your hands on your back.

1 Squeeze your buttocks and, with a straight back, lean forward to about a 45° angle. Pull your belly button in to support your back.
2 Pushing your right toe into the floor for resistance, squeeze your buttocks to return to an upright position.
3 Repeat, then switch sides.

V Squeeze

Targets your inner thighs

STARTING POSITION

Lie on your back and extend your legs straight up, feet above your hips. Open your legs in a straddle position. Place your hands along your inner thighs.

1   As you exhale, push your hands out against your thighs while you try to squeeze your legs together.
2   Close your legs, then open in a 'V' again and repeat, each time adding resistance to the movement by pushing your hands against your legs.

Step Up

Targets your butt and thighs

STARTING POSITION

Stand with your right foot flat on a high step (the higher, the harder), your left foot on the floor. Hold your bent arms above your thighs.

1   Squeeze your right buttock to straighten your right leg and raise up to step height, letting your hands rest on your thighs.
2   Hold, then lower and repeat reps on the same leg.
3   Switch sides.

HOW TO REACH YOUR GOAL WEIGHT

- Cut calories and fat and stick to an energy-giving balanced diet like the one in *Fight Fat, Fight Fatigue: Energy Makeover*.
- Train for longer than 20 minutes and pump up the intensity with longer and tougher workouts.
- Don't forget to include 4 or 5 days a week of cardio sessions. This can include cardio machines, walking, kickboxing, Spinning and aerobic classes. This will push your body to burn more calories. Hard work? Yes, but this is all-out war against flab – and you can win it!

163

INDEX

Index